ALSO BY JACOB NEEDLEMAN

*A Sense of the Cosmos:*
*The Encounter of Modern Science*
*and Ancient Truth*

*Sacred Tradition and Present Need*
(Editor, with Dennis Lewis)

*The New Religions*

*The Sword of Gnosis* (Editor)

*Being-in-the-World*

*Religion for a New Generation*
(Editor, with A. K. Bierman and James A. Gould)

# ON THE WAY
## TO
# SELF KNOWLEDGE

# ON THE WAY
# TO
# SELF KNOWLEDGE

*Edited by*

## Jacob Needleman

*and*

## Dennis Lewis

ALFRED A. KNOPF    NEW YORK    1976

THIS IS A BORZOI BOOK
PUBLISHED BY ALFRED A. KNOPF, INC.

Library of Congress Cataloging in Publication Data

Main entry under title:

On the way to self knowledge.

Bibliography: p.    Includes index.
  1. Psychotherapy—Addresses, essays, lectures.
  2. Psychiatry and religion—Addresses, essays, lectures.
  3. East and West—Addresses, essays, lectures.
  I. Needleman, Jacob.    II. Lewis, Dennis.
RC480.05 1976    150'.19'5    76-13706
ISBN 0-394-49753-8    0-394-73280-4 (pbk.)

FIRST EDITION

# Contents

# Acknowledgments

I wish to express my gratitude to the Far West Institute of San Francisco and to the Marsden Foundation of New York for the extraordinary help they provided in enabling me to organize this series of lectures and to deepen its purpose.

I wish also to thank my friends Michael and Dulce Murphy for allowing me once again to make use of the unique capabilities of Esalen Institute, and Susan Graham of the Student Union at the University of California Medical Center for her responsiveness and competence in helping with the physical arrangements.

Finally, I am grateful to my editor, Toinette Lippe, for instantly understanding the importance of this subject and supporting the preparation of this book at every juncture.

J.N.

# Preface

Although it remains a well-established fixture in our society, psychiatry has recently entered a period of great self-doubt. The past decade has witnessed a proliferation of innovations and experimental forms, which many observers take to be a sign of weakness in the whole enterprise of Western psychotherapy. A condition of widespread fragmentation now exists in this field, and even the very concept of mental illness has come under attack within the profession of psychiatry itself.

One of the most striking new developments is the tendency of many psychiatrists to make use of ideas and methods that are now entering our culture from the ancient spiritual traditions of Asia. This new movement, this new reaching out of psychiatry toward the psychological teachings of Eastern religions, was the theme of the series of lectures presented here, held during the winter and spring of 1975 at the University of California Medical Center in San Francisco. Our assumption was that the present volatile condition of psychotherapy, although surely a sign of crisis, is not necessarily a sign of weakness.

During the greater part of the twentieth century it has fallen to psychiatry, rather than to the religious institutions of the West, to bring to many modern people the question "Who am I and what is the meaning of my life?" Before the twentieth century, of course, and throughout history, man's search for meaning has been guided and renewed by the great religious traditions, only scattered fragments of which remain in the ideas, moral codes, symbols, and rites that have survived the passage of centuries. What does it mean, then, that psychiatry has begun questioning its own roots—its own identity and purpose—and is doing so, to some extent, by turning to ancient systems of self knowledge that have for thousands of years pointed mankind far beyond the ideals of what we customarily call "mental health"?

The turning toward the teachings of the ancient traditions is taking place not only in psychiatry but also in the natural sciences. This in fact was the central theme of *A Sense of the Cosmos* (Jacob Needleman, Doubleday, 1975). Readers of that book will notice that portions of the chapter devoted to psychotherapy appear again in the opening lecture of this book, and the reason for this is that while writing *A Sense of the Cosmos* the author became aware of the enormous importance of this question and the need to call forth direct responses to it from both practicing therapists and spiritual teachers. And so this series of lectures was born.

The crisis in psychiatry reflects a crisis in the lives of us all. For many of us the problem of where to turn for help and what kind of help to trust has by now become insoluble. The following, therefore, were the questions we placed before both the profession of psychiatry and those spiritual leaders from the East who are attempting to bring sacred tradition into close relationship with modern psychology. We put it in this way:

> More and more therapists are reaching out to absorb methods and concepts from the ancient religious traditions of the Orient. As a result more and more troubled people no longer know whether they need spiritual or psychiatric help or both. In the personal crisis of my life, how far can psychotherapy take me? How far do I wish to be taken? Is there a line that separates the spiritual path from therapeutic progress? What will result from the current effort of Western psychotherapists to make use of the teachings of the East—Buddhism, Hinduism, and Sufism? Can these efforts bring an expanded understanding of our human predicament, or will they result only in a reduction of the spiritual to the conventionally therapeutic? What actually

takes place in psychotherapy when seen against the
background of the vision of human nature offered by
sacred tradition?

Almost every psychiatrist or psychologist we approached,
from Erich Fromm to B. F. Skinner, confirmed the overriding
importance of this issue at the present moment in history.
More than one replied that he himself was now writing a book
or a chapter or an article on some facet of the relationship
between psychiatry and Eastern religion. In a very short time
we were even receiving unsolicited letters from therapists in
America and Europe who had heard about the planned series
and wished to take part. In selecting the actual speakers, we
were therefore faced with an embarrassment of riches. We
finally limited ourselves to a total of eight invited speakers. But
it could easily have been two or three times that number.

The response of the general public was equally powerful.
We had selected a moderate-sized lecture hall—the amphi-
theater of the University of California Medical School—that
would situate the series in the midst of the medical and
psychiatric community. Standing in a pit designed for demonstrating clinical data, the speakers found themselves looking up
at a large semicircle of over four hundred intensely quiet
people of varied backgrounds—professional clinicians, busi-
nessmen, religious leaders, housewives, and young people, a
great many of whom had come out of personal need rather
than intellectual curiosity. As one of the speakers, a man who
has lectured to large audiences throughout the world, later
said, "The energy in the room was extraordinary, as was the
demand for honesty that the audience placed upon me through
their seriousness."

This has been our second experience with the lecture series
as a form for exploring vital ideas and questions. Both in this
and in our previous series, *Sacred Tradition and Present Need*
(New York: Viking, 1975), we have all, speakers and audience

alike, verified together that something is possible through a lecture series that is usually much harder to find through the isolation of an article or a book, the self-protective conventions of an academic setting, or the zigzag of opinions, reactions, and short-lived syntheses of the colloquium. Some of us who spoke reported that we had never felt so weighed in the balance scales as in this setting. And many of us in the audience remarked on the frequent appearance in the room of an attention that helped us not only to take in more of the human being in front of us but also to try to hear within ourselves our own gut-level questions. In short, the conditions in many ways supported the search for an awareness that the great traditions, each in its own way, call the state of listening.

In editing these talks and putting them into book form, we were faced with a similar search: how to give the reader who was not present at the series a sense of the demand for openness that emerged beyond the contents of the ideas exchanged. In editing the written lectures and the record of questions and answers, we have tried to look between the lines, so to speak, in such a way so as not to interfere with the movements of meaning and energy that were actually taking place.

Of course, we still have a long way to go in making use of the lecture-series form. Having creative and thoughtful speakers is only the beginning. It requires as well that we formulate and constate questions that really touch the nerve of man's search for himself in the twentieth century and which compel a sincere response from those in a position to respond. But it also requires a great deal of serious attention to detail and a continual struggle against wishful thinking in the thousand and one physical arrangements that are necessary if such a series is to serve the fragile wish in ourselves to listen well to other people's answers as part of the search for our own question.

J.N.

D.L.

# ON THE WAY
# TO
# SELF KNOWLEDGE

# PSYCHIATRY
# AND THE SACRED

## Jacob Needleman

Modern psychiatry arose out of the vision that man must change himself and not depend for help upon an imaginary God. Over half a century ago, mainly through the insights of Freud and through the energies of those he influenced, the human psyche was wrested from the faltering hands of organized religion and was situated in the world of nature as a subject for scientific study. The cultural shock waves were enormous and long-lasting. But equal to them was the sense of hope that gradually took root throughout the Western world. To everyone, including those who offered countertheories to psychoanalysis, the main vision seemed indomitable: science, which had brought undreamt-of power over external nature, could now turn to explaining and controlling the inner world of man.

The era of psychology was born. By the end of the Second World War many of the best minds of the new generation were magnetized by a belief in this new science of the psyche. Under the conviction that a way was now open to assuage the confusion and suffering of mankind, the study of the mind became a standard course of work in American universities. The ranks of psychiatry swelled, and its message was carried to the public through the changing forms of literature, art, and educational theory. Against this juggernaut of new hope, organized religion was helpless. The concepts of human nature which had guided the Judaeo-Christian tradition for two thousand years had now to be altered and corrected just as three hundred years earlier the Christian scheme of the cosmos retreated against the onslaught of the scientific revolution. But although psychiatry in its many forms pervades our present culture, the hope it once contained has slowly ebbed away. The once charismatic psychoanalyst has become encapsulated within the workaday medical establishment, itself the object of growing public cynicism. The behaviorist who once stunned the world by defining man as a bundle of manageable reactions finds himself reduced to mere philosophizing and to the practice of piecemeal psychological cosmetics. In the burgeoning field of psychophysiology the cries of "breakthrough" echo without real conviction before the awesome and mysterious structure of the human brain. And as for experimental psychology, it has become mute; masses of data accumulated over decades of research with animals remain unrelated and seemingly unrelatable to the suffering, fear, and frustration of everyday human life.

The growing feeling of helplessness among psychiatrists and the cries for help from the masses of modern people operate in perverse contrast to the constant psychologizing of the media. Amid the "answers" provided by publications ranging in sophistication from *Reader's Digest* to *Psychology Today*, millions seem quite simply to have accepted that their lives have no great direction and ask only for help to get them through the night. The once magical promise of a transformation of the mind through psychiatry has quietly disappeared.

Of course, questions about the meaning of life and death and one's relationship to the universe may still tear at a person's insides. But now neither psychiatry nor the Church is able to respond even from the same gut level at which such questions can arise—far less from a level of universal knowledge and intuitive relationship which perceives certain cries for help as the seed of the desire for self-transformation.

No one suffers from this lack more than the psychiatrists themselves, more and more of whom despair over their inability to help other human beings in the fundamental way they once dreamed possible. Faced with the accelerating pressure of technology upon the normal patterns of human life, faced with the widespread effects of modern man's twisted relationship to nature, and yearning for a coherent purpose in living, they have come to see themselves as being in the same situation as their patients and the rest of us.

Such, in brief, is the background of a new question that is now arising concerning the hidden structure and distortions of man's inner life. Over the past decade there has taken place in our culture a widespread attraction to ideas and spiritual methods rooted in the ancient traditions of Asia and the Middle East. Starting in California, this movement initially had all the earmarks of a fad, a youthful reaction against the excesses of scientism and technocracy. This "spiritual revolution" still retains many characteristics of naïve enthusiasm. But the tendency to mobilize scattered fragments of ancient religious teachings has spread far beyond the borders of what has been called "Californialand" and is now having its effect within the very realm that scarcely a generation ago banished religion under the label of neurosis. A large and growing number of psychotherapists are now convinced that the Eastern religions offer an understanding of the mind far more complete than anything yet envisaged by Western science. At the same time, the leaders of the new religions themselves— the numerous gurus and spiritual teachers now in the West— are reformulating and adapting the traditional systems according to the language and atmosphere of modern psychology.

For example, in Berkeley, during the summers of 1973 and 1974, the Tibetan lama Tarthang Tulku led a six-week seminar in meditation exercises and Buddhist philosophy especially designed for professional psychologists. "What I mainly learned here," remarked one participant, "was how limited my concept of therapy had been. Ninety percent of what we are concerned with would be a joke to Rinpoche." * Another, a

---

* Tibetan for "teacher."

Freudian analyst from New York, left convinced that Tibetan Buddhism can reverse the "hardening of the arteries" which has afflicted the practice of psychoanalysis.

Yet another Tibetan teacher, Chögyam Trungpa, Rinpoche, is working on an even larger scale in this direction and is now establishing a psychiatric center where ancient Tibetan methods will be mingled with modern psychotherapeutic techniques. Taking his inspiration from elements of the Sufi tradition (the mystical core of the Islamic religion), psychologist Robert Ornstein writes:

> We are now for the first time in a position to begin seriously dealing with a psychology which can speak of a 'transcendence of time as we know it.' . . . These traditional psychologies have been relegated to the 'esoteric' or the 'occult,' the realm of the mysterious—the word most often employed is 'mysticism.' . . . For Western students of psychology and science, it is time to begin a new synthesis, to 'translate' some of the concepts and ideas of traditional psychologies into modern psychological terms, to regain a balance lost. To do this, we must first extend the boundaries of inquiry of modern science, *extend our concept of what is possible for man.* *

Space does not permit the mention of more than a fragment of all the activity and theorizing now taking place among psychiatrists and psychologists attracted to Zen and Tibetan Buddhism, Sufism, Hinduism in its numerous forms, and, lately, even the practices of early monastic and Eastern Christianity, as well as certain surviving remnants of the mystical Judaic tradition—Kabbalah and Hasidism. There is also the work of the humanistic and existentialist schools of psychology, pioneered by the researches of A. H. Maslow, which are converging their energies on the mystical, or, as they call it, "transpersonal," dimension of psychology. Studies of

* Robert E. Ornstein, *The Psychology of Consciousness* (San Francisco: W. H. Freeman and Company, 1972).

6

states of consciousness, peak experiences, biofeedback, the psychophysiology of yoga, and "mind-expanding" drugs are more often than not set within the context of ideas and systems that hark back to the ancient integrative sciences of man. Finally, there is the acceleration of interest in the teachings of Carl Jung, who from the very beginning moved away from the scientism of his mentor, Freud, and toward the symbols and metaphysical concepts of the esoteric and occult.

With all these disparate movements, it is no wonder that thousands of troubled men and women throughout America no longer know whether they need psychological or spiritual help. The line is blurred that divides the therapist from the spiritual guide. As one observer, speaking only half facetiously, put it: "The shrinks are beginning to sound like gurus, and the gurus are beginning to sound like shrinks."

But is it so easy to distinguish between the search for happiness and the search for transformation? Are psychotherapy and spiritual tradition simply two different approaches to the same goal, two different conceptions of what is necessary for well-being, peace of mind, and personal fulfillment? Or are they two quite separate directions that human life can take? What is the real difference between sacred tradition and psychotherapy?

Consider this fragment of an old Scottish fairy tale attributed to the pre-Christian Celts. It tells of two brothers meeting on the side of an enchanted mountain. One is climbing the mountain and the other is descending. One is being led upward by a miraculous crane, to which he is attached by a long golden thread. The other is led downward by a snarling black dog straining at an iron chain. They stop to speak about their journey and compare their difficulties. Each describes the same sorts of dangers and obstacles—precipices, huge sheer boulders, wild animals—and the same pleasures—wondrous vistas, beautiful, fragrant flowers. They agree to continue their journey together, but immediately the crane pulls the first brother upward and the dog drags the second downward. The first youth cuts the golden thread and seeks to guide himself upward solely by what he has heard from the other. But although all the obstacles are exactly as the second brother has indicated, he finds them unexpectedly guarded by evil spirits, and without the crane to guide him he is constantly driven back and is himself eventually transformed into a spirit who must eternally stand guard inside a gaping crevasse.

The larger context of this tale is not known, but it may serve very well to open the question of the relationship between psychiatry and the sacred. Of all the numerous legends, fairy tales, and myths that concern what are called "the two paths of life" (sometimes designated "the path of the fall" and "the path of the return"), this particular fragment uniquely focuses on a neglected point about the differences between the obstacles to awakening and the obstacles to happiness. The tale is saying that however similar the obstacles to these two aims might appear, in actuality they are very different. And woe to him who fails to take into account both possible movements of the inner life of man. Woe to him who does not attend to both the divinity and the animal in himself. He will never move either toward "earthly happiness" *or* toward self-transformation.

This tale almost seems specifically designed to expose our present uncertainty about so-called "spiritual psychology." Consider the ideas emanating from ancient Eastern traditions, that are now entering into the stream of modern psychological language: ideas about "states of consciousness," "enlightenment," "meditation," "freedom from the ego," "self-realization"—to name only a few. Is it possible that each of these terms can be understood from two different angles of vision? For example, does one meditate in order to resolve the problems of life or to become conscious of the automatic movement of forces in oneself?

Our question concerns psychiatry considered as a means to an end, as the removal of obstacles that stand in the way of happiness. (I choose the word *happiness* only for the sake of brevity; we could equally well speak of the goal of psychiatry as useful living, the ability to stand on one's own feet, or adjustment to society.) These obstacles to happiness—our fears, unfulfilled desires, violent emotions, frustrations, maladaptive behavior—are the "sins" of our modern psychiatric "religion." But now we are asked to understand that there exist teachings about the universe and about man under whose guidance the psychological obstacles, these "sins against happiness," may be accepted and studied as material for the development of the force of consciousness.

Perhaps at this point it would be helpful to pause briefly and reflect upon the general idea of the transmutation of consciousness. The word *consciousness* is used nowadays in so many different senses that it is tempting to single out one or another aspect of consciousness as its primary characteristic. The difficulty is compounded by the fact that our attitude toward knowledge about ourselves is like our attitude toward new discoveries about the external world. We so easily lose our balance when something extraordinary is discovered in science or when we come upon an exciting new explanatory concept: immediately the whole machinery of systematic thought comes into play. Enthusiasm sets in, accompanied by a proliferation of utilitarian explanations, which then stand in the way of direct encounters with the real, moving world.

In a like manner, a new experience of the self tempts us to believe we have discovered the sole direction for the development of consciousness, aliveness, or—as it is sometimes called—presence. The same machinery of explanatory thought comes into play, accompanied by pragmatic programs for "action." It is not only followers of the new religions who may fall victim to this tendency, taking fragments of traditional teachings which have brought them a new experience of themselves and building a religion around them. This tendency in ourselves also accounts for much of the fragmentation of modern psychology, just as it accounts for fragmentation in the natural sciences.

9

In order to call attention to this tendency in ourselves, the traditional teachings—as in the Bhagavad Gita, for example— make a fundamental distinction between *consciousness* and the *contents of consciousness.* In the light of this distinction, everything we ordinarily take to be consciousness (or our real self) is actually identified as the *contents of consciousness:* our perceptions of things, our sense of personal identity, our emotions, and our thoughts in all their colors and gradations.

This ancient distinction has two crucial messages for us. On the one hand, it tells us that what we feel to be the best of ourselves as human beings is only part of a total structure containing layers of mind, feeling, and sensation far more active, subtle, and unifying than what we have settled for as our best. These layers are incredibly numerous and need to be peeled back, as it were, one by one along the path of inner growth (the "upward path" of our tale) until one touches in oneself the fundamental intelligent force in the cosmos.

At the same time, this distinction also communicates that the awakening of consciousness requires a constant effort. It is telling us that anything in ourselves, no matter how subtle, fine, or intelligent, no matter how close to reality or virtuous, no matter how still or violent—any action, any thought, any intuition or experience—immediately devours our attention and becomes automatically transformed into *contents,* around which gather all the opinions, feelings, and distorted sensations that are the supports of our secondhand sense of identity. In short, we are told that the evolution of man is always (eternally) "vertical" to the downward-flowing stream of mental, emotional, and physical associations within the human psyche. The downward "pull of gravity" is within ourselves. And seen in this light, there are no concentric layers of human awareness that need to be peeled back like the skins of an onion, but only one skin, one veil, that is constantly forming regardless of the quality of the psychic field at any given moment.

From this latter perspective, the main requirement for

understanding the nature of consciousness is the repeated *effort* to be aware of whatever is taking place in the whole of ourselves at any given moment. All definitions or systematic explanations, no matter how profound, are secondary. Thus teachings about consciousness, both of the ancient masters and of modern psychologists, can be a distraction if they are presented to us in a way that does not support the effort to be aware of the totality of ourselves in the present moment.

In traditional cultures special terms surround this quality of self knowledge, connecting it to the direct human participation in a higher, all-encompassing reality, "beyond the Earth," as it is sometimes said. The existence of these special terms, such as *satori* (Zen Buddhism), *fana* (Islam), *pneuma* (Christianity), and many others, may serve for us as a sign that this effort of total awareness was always set apart from the normal, everyday goods of organized social life. And while the traditional teachings tell us that any human being may engage in the search for this quality of presence, it is ultimately recognized that only very few will actually wish to do so, for it is a struggle that in the last analysis is undertaken solely for its own sake, without recognizable psychological motivation. And so, imbedded within every traditional culture there is said to be an "esoteric" or inner path discoverable only by those who yearn for something inexplicably beyond the duties and satisfactions of religious, intellectual, moral, and social life.

What we can recognize as psychiatric methods in traditional cultures must surely be understood in this light. Psychosis and neurosis were obviously known to the ancient world just as they are known in the few remaining traditional societies that still exist today in scattered pockets throughout the world. In a traditional culture, then, the challenge of what we would call psychotherapy consisted in bringing a person back to a normal life without stamping out the nascent impulse toward transformation in the process of treatment. To do this, a practitioner would have had to recognize the difference in a man between thwarted normal psychological functioning and the unsatisfied yearning ("that comes from nowhere," as one Sufi teacher has described it) for the evolution of consciousness. Certainly, that is one reason why traditionally the "psychotic" was treated by the priest. It is probably also why what we would call "neurosis" was handled within the once-intact family structure, permeated as this structure was by the religious teachings of the culture.

It has been observed that modern psychiatry could have assumed its current place only after the breakdown of the patriarchal family structure that dates back to the beginnings of recorded history. But the modern psychiatrist faces a tremendously difficult task as a surrogate parent even beyond the problems that have been so thoroughly described under the psychoanalytic concept of transference. For there may be something far deeper, subtler, and more intensely human, something that echoes of a "cosmic dimension," hidden behind the difficulties and therapeutic opportunities of the classical psychoanalytic transference situation. We have already given this hidden "something" a name: the desire for self-transformation. In the ancient patriarchal family structure (as I am told it still exists, for example, among the Brahmin families of India) the problems of living a normal, fulfilled life are never separated from the sense of a higher dimension of human existence. What we might recognize as therapeutic counseling is given by family members or friends, but in such a way that a troubled individual will never confuse the two possible directions that his life can take. He is helped to see that the obstacles to happiness are not necessarily the obstacles to "spiritual realization," as it is called in such traditions. A great many of what we take to be intolerable restrictions—such as predetermined marriage partners or vocations—are connected to this spiritual factor in the make-up of the traditional patterns of family life.

Can the modern psychiatrist duplicate this aspect of family influence? Almost certainly, he cannot. For one thing, he himself probably did not grow up in such a family milieu; almost none of us in the modern world have. Therefore, the task he faces is even more demanding than most of us realize. He may recognize that religion has become a destructive influence in people's lives because the Path of transformation offered by the traditions has become covered over by ideas and doctrines we have neither understood nor experienced. He may even see that this same process of getting lost in undigested spiritual ideas and methods is taking place among many followers of the new religions. But at the same time, perhaps he sees that there can exist in people—be they neurotic or normal—this hidden desire for inner evolution. How can the patient be led to a normal, happy life without crushing this other, hidden impulse that can bring human life into a radically different dimension—whether or not a person ever becomes happy or self-sufficient or adjusted in the usual sense of these words? For the development of consciousness in man may not necessarily entail the development of what would be called a "normal," "well-adjusted," or "self-sufficient" personality.

Let us now look more closely at the process of modern psychotherapeutic healing against the background of the ancient, traditional understanding of human nature.

We may begin with the idea of levels of unity within the human organism. Both the spiritual guide and the therapist come upon the individual existing in a state of hidden fragmentation and dispersal. A man cannot be what he wishes to be. His behavior, his feelings, his very thoughts bring him pain or, what is even worse, an endless round of empty satisfactions and unconfronted terrors. As it is said, "he does not know who he is." The sense of identity that society and his upbringing have thrust upon him does not square with what he feels to be his instincts, his gut-level needs, and his deepest aspirations. He is constantly fleeing from loneliness or boredom, states in which there is nothing or no one to confirm his identity through the stimulation of desire.

Beneath the fragile sense of personal identity, the individual is actually an innumerable swarm of disconnected impulses, thoughts, reactions, opinions, and sensations, which are triggered into activity by causes of which he is totally unaware. Yet at each moment, the individual identifies himself with whichever of this swarm of impulses and reactions happens to be active, automatically affirming each as "himself," and then taking a stand either for or against this "self," depending on the particular pressures that the social environment has brought to bear upon him since his childhood.

The traditions identify this affirming-and-denying process as the real source of human misery and the chief obstacle to the development of man's inherent possibilities. Through this affirmation and denial a sort of form is constructed around each of the passing impulses originating in the different parts of the human organism. And this continuous, unconscious affirmation of identity traps a definite amount of precious psychic energy in a kind of encysting process that is as much chemical-biological as it is psychological. The very nerves and muscles of the body are called to defend and support the affirmation of "I" around each of the countless groups of impulses and reactions as they are activated.

Several years ago, when I was moderating a seminar of psychiatrists and clinicians, the real dimensions of this affirmation process were brought home in a very simple and powerful way. We were all discussing the use of hypnosis in therapy, and the question arose as to what actually takes place in hypnosis, and what it means that human beings are in general hypnotizable. At some point during the discussion one of the participants began to speak in a manner that riveted everyone's attention. He was a psychoanalyst, the oldest and most respected member present.

"Only once in my life," he said, "did I ever use hypnosis with a patient. It was in the Second World War, when I was in the Swiss Army. There was this poor soldier in front of me, and for some reason I decided to test whether or not he would be susceptible to posthypnotic suggestion. I easily brought him into a trance and, simply by way of experiment, I suggested to him that after he awoke he would stamp his foot three times whenever I snapped my fingers. All perfectly standard procedure. After I brought him out of the trance state and we spoke for a while, I dismissed him, and just as he was leaving the room I snapped my fingers. He immediately responded and stamped his foot according to the suggestion. 'Wait a minute,' I shouted. 'Tell me, why did you stamp your foot?' His face suddenly turned beet red. 'Damn it all,' he said, 'I've got something in my shoe.' "

The speaker slowly puffed on his pipe and his face became extremely serious. The rest of us could not understand why he seemed to be making so much of this well-known phenomenon of posthypnotic fabrication. But he maintained his silence, staring somberly down the length of his pipe. No one else said a word—it was obvious that he was trying to formulate something that he took to be quite important. Then, with his face suddenly as open as a child's, he looked up at me, and said:

"Do you think the whole of our psychic life is like that?"

A strange and rather awkward silence followed. Some of the company obviously felt that this man, whom everyone acknowledged as a great practitioner, was having a temporary intellectual lapse. But the others, myself included, were struck by the extraordinary feeling he had put into this simple question, as though he were at that very moment internally revising everything he had ever understood about the mind.

Everyone was looking at me, waiting for me to reply. And, in fact, what he was driving at had already dawned on me. But before I could speak, he went on in exactly the same way except that his face now registered not only amazement, but something akin to horror:

"Do you think," he said, "that every movement we make, every word we say, every thought we have is like that? Could it be that we are always 'fabricating' in a sort of low-grade posthypnotic haze? Because there's one thing I am sure of, though only now do I see its importance: the moment I asked that soldier why he had stamped his foot, there was a split second when he realized that *he* had not *done* anything at all. A moment when he realized that the fact was simply that his foot stamped the ground 'all by itself.' By asking him why he had stamped his foot, I was in effect suggesting to his mind that *he* had *done* something. In short, I was still hypnotizing him—or, rather, I was playing into the general process of hypnosis that is going on all the time with all of us from the cradle to the grave. The contradiction made him blush, and the true facts about the foot-stamping were blotted out of awareness."

Another silence, very brief. Some of the other participants were nearly bursting with impatience to have their say. But I chose not to recognize anyone else. I was totally fascinated with where the thought of this speaker was taking him. He went on for quite a while, weaving his speculations around the possibility that the whole of man's psychic life is the product of suggestions coming from different sources, some immediately external and others stored in the mechanisms of memory. And this whole process, he concluded, is constantly screened from our awareness by the belief, also conditioned into us, that we are acting, individual selves. Our so-called "freedom of the will" is only an *ex post facto* identification with processes that are taking place "all by themselves."

From earlier conversations with this psychiatrist, I knew he had never gone very deeply into the study of spiritual traditions, not even Western traditions. He knew nothing about the Buddhist diagnosis of the human condition as permeated by the delusion of selfhood. He was totally unfamiliar with the ancient Pythagorean symbolism of reincarnation. In that symbolism the psyche (or soul) that does not progress toward the evolution of consciousness is said to reincarnate into lower forms of life (such as animals). As in the Buddhist teaching, this image of reincarnation symbolizes the prison of identifying with partial and automatic psychic processes, to the extent that the whole energy of the psyche is more and more "encysted" or trapped within a narrow range of psychological postures, repeating over and over again, for "endless eons."

What, then, is the picture we have before us?

Through social custom, through education, through the indoctrinations and influences of religion, art, and family, the individual is made to accept at a very early age that he is an integral whole, persisting through time, possessing a real identity and a definite psychic structure. Yet as an adult, he is actually a thousand loosely connected psychophysical "cysts." As he leaves childhood and affirms this socially conditioned identity, he is actually leaving behind the possible growth of his inner structure. The evolution of a true psychic integrity comes to a halt, requiring, as it does, the very energy that is now diverted and consumed in upholding the sense of "I." The individual becomes a lie, a lie that is now ingrained in the very neural pathways of the organism. He habitually, automatically pretends he is one and whole—it is demanded of him and he demands it of himself. Yet in fact he is scattered and multiple.

But he cannot help himself now. It is useless to throw moral imperatives at him. For there is no "ruling principle" within him and thus nothing that could change the course of his inner condition. All the knowledge, experience, and impressions that are meant to nourish the development of the inner psychic structure with which he was born are either sloughed off and "grounded," or absorbed in distorted fashion solely to support the hidden affirmation process. A man lives in his own world, as it is said. The sensitive current of feeling that is meant to permeate the entire being as an indispensable organ of knowledge and will is now channeled instead into the "emotions" of the ego—such as fear, self-satisfaction, self-pity, and competitiveness. Blended with the extremely volatile and combinative energies of sex, these emotions become so pervasive that they are accepted as the real nature of man, as his "unconscious" or his "animal nature," the reality behind the appearances.

And it is true. These emotions and drives, now fueled and maintained by stealing the energies of the sexual nature, are pervasive and all-powerful. And yet, in a deeper sense, it is not true. For these emotions are only powerful in the formation and maintenance of the affirmation-and-negation process that screens the basic fragmentation of the human psyche. In the traditional understanding, the real unconscious is the hidden psychic integrity, which has been forgotten and left behind in childhood, and which requires for its development not egoistic satisfactions, not "recognition from others," not sexual or libidinal pleasure, not even physical security, food, and shelter. This "original face" of man requires only the energy of truth—that is to say, the real impressions of the external and internal world carried to the embryonic essence of man by means of the faculty of free attention. Thus, according to tradition, there is something potentially divine within man, which is born when his physical body is born but which needs for its growth an entirely different sustenance from what is needed by the physical body or the social self.

Traditionally, then, the term *self knowledge* has an extraordinary meaning. It is neither the acquisition of information about oneself nor a deeply felt insight nor moments of recognition against the ground of psychological theory. It is an act that is in itself the principal means by which the evolving part of man can be nourished with an energy that is as real, or more so, as the energy delivered to the physical organism by the food we eat. Thus it is not a question of acquiring strength, independence, self-esteem, security, "meaningful relationships," or any of the other goods upon which the social order is based and which have been identified as the components of psychological health. It is solely a matter of digesting deep impressions of myself as I actually am from moment to moment: a disconnected, helpless collection of impulses and reactions, a being of disharmonized mind, feeling, and instinct.


I should like to conclude by asking my question from a slightly different angle. Both among psychiatrists and the general public a widespread sense of crisis has set in concerning the psychological condition of man on this planet. Accelerated changes in the patterns of social life and the threats of war and overdeveloped technology are now more and more being met by the unleashing of powerful ideas torn from the traditional integrative sciences of man, against the background of the swift modernization of traditional cultural environments throughout the world. The mixture of these forces has induced a combination of fear and a visionary mentality concerning the possible evolution of planetary and individual man.

Yet in the private lives of almost everyone these same forces of scientific advance and cultural homogenization continue to produce painful and dehumanizing effects on the quality of our lived experience. The passive acceptance of scientific concepts of time, space, energy—and lately of mind—drives man further and further away from discovering his own space, his own time, his own vital energy, and his own active intelligence. So connected to the species has the individual become that his patterns of thought and feeling are now dictated on a world-wide basis by the needs and sufferings of the biological organism, man-on-earth.

Lost in all this is the human middle zone between the creature of earth and the private universe called "atman" in the Hindu traditions, "spirit" in Christianity, or simply "myself," "I," my original face. This middle zone of human life was once known as the family, the community, the tribe. Through the conditions of family life, the development and interiorization of the self could take place alongside the growth of the individual as a cell in the body of man-on-earth. The middle zone of human life was the product of a religion in which both heaven and earth, as ideas and as possible dimensions of living, could be the everyday environment of human life. The exaggerated influence of scientism destroyed this two-natured environment quite as decisively as it now threatens to destroy the environment of biological man. Against this former, more fundamental environmental destruction, modern psychiatry arose to help bring man back into contact with the life of feeling, a life that at the turn of the century was already being obliterated by dogmatic, intercultural religion, religion also cut off from the middle zone of human life, religion become worldly in the sense of being homogeneous, doctrinaire, and explanatory. In international Christianity, the Church lost contact with the hidden existence in man of an embryonic yearning for the eternal and instead imposed beliefs and explanatory concepts patterned after the species-and-survival knowledge of modern science. In the present era the centuries-long process was completed by which the Christian religion surrendered its ancient quiet influence on the heart of man and gave itself up instead to persuading, arguing, and compelling radical choices on a being in whom the decision to seek for oneself does not have to be *made* but only *heard.*

In the nineteenth and twentieth centuries the concept of mysticism was developed in order to classify a part of the self that science could not explain. Later, the same forces that classified mysticism eventually defined the mind, and, as we have said, the mind became an object of scientific exploration. Mysticism was pushed even further aside while the mind as a whole was naturalized—that is, understood as part of the biological organism. That there is such a mind, which functions as part of the biological organism, was always known and given various names in the traditional teachings; disturbances of this physical, biological mind, the species mind, were always treated by the traditional physician-priests, whose task it was to distinguish the sufferings of the physical mind from the yearnings for growth that emanated from the private mind, or soul.

Today, however, with the influx of fragments of traditional teachings and with the current disillusionment in the sciences, techniques for treating the physical mind of man are being joined without real guidance to ideas and methods that pertain to the individual, private mind that was always understood to be rooted in another level of reality—a mind, a consciousness, that is said to have a life independent of the motivations that constitute the ego of the human being.

At the heart of the great traditions is the idea that the search for truth is undertaken for its own sake ultimately. These traditional teachings in their entirety propose to show man the nature of this search and the laws behind it—laws which, as I have suggested, too often get lost in our enthusiasm for ideas and explanations that we have not deeply absorbed in the fire of living with all its suffering and confusion. Psychotherapy, on the other hand, is surely a *means* to an end—to the goal we have called happiness. Unlike the way offered by tradition, therapy is never an end in itself, never a way of life, but is motivated toward a goal that the therapist sees more clearly than his patient. The therapist may even experiment with invented methods to achieve this goal and often succeeds. But is it recognized that two kinds of success are possible in the process of therapy? On the one hand, the successful result may be a patient in whom the wish for evolution has been totally "disillusioned" and stamped out through the deliberate arousal in himself of the very quality of egoistic emotion which the traditions seek to break down and dissolve. But another kind of success may be possible in certain cases—a patient in whom the wish for evolution has been driven inside, who no longer dreams of a response to this wish from the outside world, but who now has within him an even greater sensitivity and hunger for deeper contact with himself. To the outside observer, such a person may seem to have developed a certain "inner-directedness," but in actuality he is precisely the sort of person who may desperately need what the traditions seek to communicate. The effort of contemporary teachers from the East to bring their message to such people in terms that are neither freighted with dead antiquity nor compromised by modern psychologisms constitutes the real spiritual drama of the present age.

I suspect that psychiatrists sense there can be these two different kinds of success in the process of psychotherapy. But the second class of patients probably leave the therapist before the treatment is far advanced, while the first class of patients stay in treatment as long as they can. Therefore, this second type of patient is probably not consciously or officially recognized by the profession of psychiatry.

So the question comes to this: in the personal crisis of my life, what sort of help do I seek? And the answer, in all sincerity, seems to revolve around the following fact. It is in the periods *between* crises that I reflect upon different paths and set up standards regarding whom I will trust and who has the truth about human nature. The point is that when I am in trouble it is not the spiritual guide or psychotherapist that I turn to. It is something in myself, a part of myself, that I turn to. Some ideas, some habits of thinking, some memories, some reports settled in my mind, some emotional associations: these are the guides that lead me to you. In the moment when life is crushing me, it may seem that I take any hand that is offered. But it is not true. I have an "inner guide" that leads me to you.

Of course, it is extremely inaccurate to refer to this collection of chance associations and emotional impulses, this loose federation of fears, prejudices, and habitual patterns of self-suggestion, as an inner guide. It is an inaccurate phrase if by "guide" we mean someone or something that leads us to the truth about ourselves. For, this "inner guide" knows nothing of truth. Moreover, it gives great-sounding names—such as "transformation," "freedom," and "self-expression"—only to experiences that conform to its chance requirements, its need for the illusion of unity, while the rest of my nature remains unknown and unintegrated. This "inner guide" is the ego. Yet the term *inner guide* is accurate in that it is actually what I turn to when facing both sacred tradition and psychotherapy. It is what gets me through the night, and through my life.

Which of you, spiritual guides and psychotherapists, knows this aspect of my nature and its real place in my life? Which of you takes it into account when I ask for help? Which of you can hear the faint cry behind it of something in myself that wishes for truth? And which of you can address both sides of my nature, these two sides that we are told are created in man to struggle with each other so that out of this struggle a new being, a real *I*, can be born. For the "third brother"—so the traditions tell us—can only come into being and move forward out of the struggle between the other two.

I see, therefore, that in the last analysis the names "spiritual guide" and "psychotherapist" are not the essential thing. I see that even the ideas and methods offered me by a spiritual teacher can be taken over by my egoistic "inner guide" and used to take me only toward the lesser unities of social happiness and independence. And what of the help offered me under the name of psychotherapy? Among you therapists, do there exist people who feel the two sides of human nature and are sensitive to their simultaneous claims, the possible struggle between them, the emergence within man of that middle world between heaven and earth in which—classically speaking, and using the ancient language of alchemy—good and evil, active and passive, masculine and feminine engage in a warfare that can discover the moment of internal love, an inner exchange of substance leading to the birth of the New Man?

Spiritual guides and psychotherapists, what do your names mean? How should we accept what you call yourselves? Behind these names, which of you are the real spiritual guides and which the real psychotherapists? We need to know. I need to know.

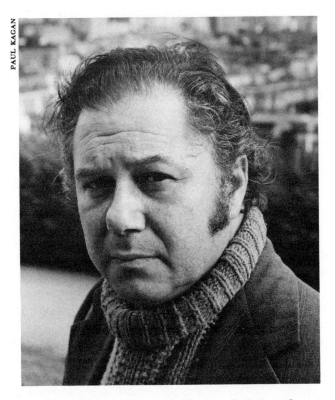

*Jacob Needleman, Ph.D.,* Professor of Philosophy at San Francisco State University, is author of *Being-in-the-World, The New Religions,* and *A Sense of the Cosmos: The Encounter of Modern Science and Ancient Truth.* Coeditor of *Sacred Tradition and Present Need,* he has written in the field of philosophy, comparative religion, and psychology, examining both ancient and contemporary forms of man's perennial search for himself.

*Dennis Lewis,* coeditor of *Sacred Tradition and Present Need,* is a free-lance writer and editor living in San Francisco.

# THE CHRISTIAN
# SACRED TRADITION
# AND PSYCHOTHERAPY

## Thomas P. Malone

Our culture appears finally to have captured its native sacred tradition. Much of the lamentable and destructive stagnation (and apathy) of our society since the turn of the century can be attributed to the escalating institutionalization of our sacred traditions. For, together with art, the spiritual traditions of a people are its primary resource for cultural change, intellectual replenishment, and creative leadership.

Institutionalized to the point where it becomes mainly a conservatory for the consensual secular values of the culture, the religious impulse in man eventually seeks other expressions and different prophets. Therefore, it is not at all surprising that Eastern traditions have been imported in all of their exciting and exotic varieties. For better or worse these Eastern teachings have gradually attached themselves to our psychological disciplines. It is true that the majority of "scientists" in the behavioral field are somewhat disturbed by this unwelcome association. Some are outraged at the notion that Zen Buddhism may offer a more workable theoretical basis for personal growth and change than behaviorism. Others are politely embarrassed, much as they were when telepathy and psychokinesis intruded as serious subjects for research. Nonetheless, a significant and impressive minority of psychologists are welcoming these strange and exotic influences and are seriously attempting to integrate them into their psychotherapeutic systems.

I am of that minority who are impressed with much of the pregnant wisdom of these alien teachings, but at the same time I feel a prior commitment. And I hope to show here that our Christian tradition divested of its institutionalized armor is as exciting and as facilitative of human growth as Zen Buddhism or Sufism—this despite the fact that the Christian tradition often presents itself in psychotherapy as the main supportive system for the defenses of patients.*

In his introductory talk Dr. Needleman asks with a great deal of feeling: "Spiritual guides and psychotherapists, what do your names mean? How should we accept what you call yourselves? Behind these names, which of you are the real spiritual guides and which the real psychotherapists? We need to know. I need to know."

Now, over the years it has struck me as curious that although we have managed to develop a basic theory of man's physical evolution, and although we have resolutely pursued a more adequate understanding of the evolution of the physical universe, we have not at all studied the evolution of the human spirit—Jung being the most outstanding exception. Why the conspiracy of avoidance and apathy concerning evolution of human personhood? Does consciousness abhor scrutiny of itself? Does it insist on some sort of untouchable self-reverence? Are we still rat-oriented because of our embarrassment at the nineteenth-century introspectionists? And are we still

---

* In fact, the institutionalized Christian ethic has been covertly integrated into our traditional orthodox and conventional psychological scientisms. Behavioral-modification theory appears especially to contain almost intact the institutionalized Christian tradition. It is based totally on an ethic of good-and-evil, reward-and-punishment, and heaven-and-hell dynamics. God exists outside the person, and although presented as the wise benevolent secular big brother, the behavioral modifier is nonetheless the Calvinistic omnipotent punitive and rewarding God. The original Christian tradition spoke more of love, grace, acceptance, relationship, surrender, God in man, and many of the basic postulates of Eastern sacred traditions.

currying the condescending nod of reluctant approval from the "real scientists"? Do we continue to believe that only by unraveling the human brain can we ever illuminate the mysteries of how consciousness and the human spirit have evolved? The notion that the soul can evolve may be uncomprehensible, or even blasphemous to some. But if the soul does not evolve, it would clearly be the only form of life that does not. I am convinced that man's soulness *has* evolved, and will continue to evolve, provided we sufficiently value those psychological mutants called patients, who are the vehicles of that evolution.

There is a conversation in T. S. Eliot's *The Cocktail Party* in which Dr. Reilly, the psychiatrist, is discussing with Celia what happens in psychiatric treatment. Celia anxiously inquires about the possible outcomes of therapy, and Dr. Reilly carefully explains that for most patients therapy has little risk. They are concerned with adjustment or with correcting defects in their personal development. These persons may or may not be helped, or redeemed. Most often they can return to their communities as effective players.

But there are other so-called patients who search not for adjustment to their history or community, but for an expanded humanness. As Dr. Reilly points out, this search is fraught with danger, since it is possible that the journey may end in complete alienation: human beings pointlessly wandering through an asylum, weaving and spinning the dreams and aspirations of the human spirit. It is as if the fictional Dr. Reilly anticipated the likes of Ronnie Laing, who has made the outlandish suggestion that the crazies of this world are those willing to explore the inner world of man's spirit to find more soul, spirit, or humanity. And if they fail, as most do, they become like the saber-toothed tigers—beautiful, pitiful mutants doomed to a deviant, uncreative extinction.

This has been my experience as a psychotherapist. Most of my patients are indeed patients in the ordinary medical sense of the word. They seek adjustments either to their history or their community. They seek healing, and this is surely a legitimate goal. But occasionally, and more often in recent years, I encounter patients who are not at all patients in the ordinary medical sense. They do not seek healing, and adjustment seems to be the least of their concerns. It is a rather eerie experience—as if you are in the presence of someone not content to be content. They appear to be driven to more humanity, more soul, toward a kind of spiritual explosion. Driven, but not in the usual sense of compulsiveness. I have come to see these fortunate or unfortunate persons as psychological or spiritual mutants who carry, usually unwillingly, the responsibility for the evolution of the human spirit. My impression is that these mutants cannot be identified by whether they are "healthy people" searching for growth in psychotherapy or crazies and depressed people. Any single person in either group can be committed to either adjustment or spiritual evolution. It has less to do with the manner in which the person presents himself than with the characterological intent of that person.

These people obviously are very special and should be valued as such. They are important to humanity, probably more important than Arafat or Kissinger or even Catfish Hunter. Precious as they are, to whom should they be entrusted—psychotherapists or spiritual guides? Dr. Needleman's question. I think it depends on who are the *real* psychotherapists. His question. And my answer:

I am a psychotherapist by training, by profession, and, most important, by virtue of special developmental experiences in my early life leading to formation of my character structure. That particular character structure sharply limited my vocational choices. I tried being an artist. I tried being a priest, but since the Church at the time had serious difficulties with celibacy, I couldn't. I tried one year of law school but was so confused by its vacuum of values that in retrospect I concluded I had gone beyond the boundaries of my characterological territory. I then began my training in psychotherapy. I could have become a kindergarten teacher, a football coach, maybe even a certain kind of bartender or even a neighborhood cop. There are many varieties of secular priests. My character required me to continue the work begun as a child in my family, namely to maintain and nurture other persons, or, to put it more broadly: passionately to attend the human spirit. This was not at all altruistic but rather a compelling and inevitable consequence of my basic training, fairly complete in mid-adolescence.

So I describe a psychotherapist as one who by virtue of character development, subsequently implemented by a variety of trainings and practicings, passionately attends the human spirit. This may strike you as a naïve or arrogant definition, but it has the heuristic value of any operational definition. A psychotherapist *is* what I am, and psychotherapy *is* what I do. I of course am not unique or even unusual. There are many psychotherapists who are what I am and who do what I do. This despite the fact that our personalities are often quite dissimilar, and certainly our behavior—our techniques in doing psychotherapy—differs enormously.

Are you then a psychotherapist by virtue of your training, because society so certifies you? Or are you a psychotherapist because you genuinely feel you are a therapeutic person, certification be damned? It depends.

Psychotherapy in its broadest sense could include all intentional action of a person or persons aimed at altering the behavior or attitudes of others. Defined so, psychotherapy would encompass education, advertising, and propaganda of every sort. It would even include bringing up children. This may sound absurdly general, but in truth it is the only definition of psychotherapy that would include everything that proceeds under that name in schools, prisons, or hospitals throughout America.

But unless it is to become as vague a term as *patriotism*, psychotherapy deserves a more dignified and limited meaning. At the very least it should include as essential the *contractual intent* of the so-called patient to enter the relationship for purposes of either help or growth. Beyond that—and speaking realistically rather than legalistically—it is difficult at the present time to isolate any other defining criteria; certainly not any commonalities of procedure or technique, and certainly not the training or professionalism of the psychotherapist. Even with that limitation, psychotherapy covers an unbelievable panorama of experiences, techniques, and gurus.

There are as many psychotherapies as there are religions: psychoanalysis, existential therapy, experiential therapy, rational-emotive therapy, behavioral modification, Gestalt, transactional analysis, supportive, eclectic, and, as the King said to Anna, et cetera, et cetera, et cetera. This is only the beginning; you can then range into psychiatric social work, counseling, education counseling, marital counseling, industrial and management consulting—then through myriad group therapies from the rigors of Slavson through the fantastics of Esalen. And still you have only touched the respectable and well-dressed cousins. You have now to cruise through the paraprofessionals, the religious, the semi- and pseudo-religious, to the commercials and the quacks. And unless you are captured by your own pomposity, you had best reserve judgment on the efficacy of any particular therapeutic experience for any particular searcher. You may be terribly wrong, even about the quacks.

In the midst of such chaos who is to say safely which are the real psychotherapists? The answer, of course, is that the real psychotherapist is the person who in fact facilitates the quest of the patient. And at this point an honest impartial observer would have to agree that there appear to be real psychotherapists in practically every sect, both orthodox and deviant, of the broad spectrum of people-nourishers. If this be true, and I am convinced it is, then the emphasis shifts from what the psychotherapist does to what the psychotherapist is—that is, his character structure, and also, although it is less important in this context, his personality. His personality is less important since it is implemental to character and so more closely allied with mere technique.

Are psychotherapists then born, as prophets were traditionally said to be born? Not at all. But I do believe psychotherapists are grown, cultivated, and raised, as I believe prophets were. Moreover, this cultivation takes a lifetime; professional training is insufficient, although very necessary (much as there is little freedom without disciplined ritual).

Before I can discuss the relationship between the sacred and psychotherapy, one further discrimination has to be made. Patients come to be healed or to grow, to seek help or ask you to journey with them in inner space, to find a happier adjustment to their history or community or to forgo comfort and happiness in order to explore the growing edges of the human spirit. Psychotherapists—and all are psychotherapists who facilitate either task—are not equally capable of relating to these two broad groups of patients. I, for example, can help the explorers much more effectively than I can those who seek healing. I have colleagues who are much more effective as healers.

The difference? I am not sure. But I do have a very private classification of psychotherapists that does not have official credentials, but which has been helpful to me in understanding my colleagues. Looked at characterologically, therapists appear to fall into one of three categories: charismatic, methodical, or natural.

*Charisma* comes from the Greek, meaning "full of the spirit," or "anointed." *Method* comes from the Greek *hodos*, meaning "a way, a road, a means of doing something" (or coming to something), and from *meta*, meaning "after"—the combined word meaning "a way after," or "coming after someone." *Natural* comes from the Latin *nasei*, meaning "to be born," or *natalis*, meaning "of birth." An interesting derivative word of "natural" is "naïve." It comes from the same primary etymon.

Charismatic therapists are full of the spirit, and their

effectiveness involves the transfer of that human spirit to their patients. It would be unfair to think of them simply as inspirational or revivalistic. Such transfer of spirit can be transforming of others, can facilitate the healing of particular life-historical wounds, and can occasionally provide another with the courage to explore the frontiers of selfhood. But when the charismatic therapist goes with a patient into the inner spaces of the human spirit, he most often leads him rather than follows or accompanies him.

Methodical therapists have a *way,* a means of doing something, and literally come after their patients. They are probably the best healers, and I suspect that as the sophistication of their means or ways continues to grow, they will become by far the most efficacious of healers. They either avoid or are ill-equipped for exploration of the human spirit. Their forte is the familiar, and the familiar (or "family-like") is the nucleus of all adjustment, either to one's history or to one's community.

The natural therapist is birth-oriented. Consequently he is interested in creation, the new rather than the renewed, impregnation, relationship, discovery, evolving life. In general, the natural therapist has interests and talents that dispose him toward the exploration of the cutting edge of human experience. You would expect him to do better with those patients who appear never content to be content. In contrast to the charismatic therapist, he searches for the spirit *in* the patient and seems most adept at providing a nourishing relationship within which that spirit or consciousness can grow or create more of itself. He walks with, even follows, but seldom leads.

I have found therapists fitting into each of these categories in practically every school of psychotherapy.


This series concerns itself with psychotherapy and the sacred. Some discriminations appeared necessary to me both regarding patients and their intent in psychotherapy, and regarding psychotherapists and the nature of their personal participation in psychotherapy. Now if we confine ourselves to that important minority of patients whose intent is growth, exploration rather than adjustment and comfort, and to those therapists whom I have termed natural therapists, and finally to the quality of the interaction between the two, then I feel we are dealing with the most significant interface of psychotherapy and the sacred.

The most immediate sacred tradition available to me is the Western Judaeo-Christian tradition. Since I am not at all expert in comparative religion or philosophy, I have chosen four of the most central concepts in the Christian tradition as a point of departure. These are: God, sin, grace, and salvation.

My intent is simply to describe these elements of "sacred tradition" as they have repeatedly emerged in my professional experience. They became part of the therapeutic dialogue for two reasons. My patients all come to me imbued with this Judaeo-Christian tradition even though most of them have long since despaired of finding nourishment for their personal search in organized religion. And these ancient words and concepts inevitably invade the dialogue—not simply because these are the words and ideas of their childhood religious experience but also because the two most suitable languages of psychotherapy are the language of the street and the language of the sacred and prophetic. The street language suffices until the therapeutic experience becomes tenderly loving, or mystical; then koan, parable, or symbol emerges out of the deep recesses of the patient's early religious experience. Not his training—his experience.

Since most of us were raised within this particular sacred tradition, I will not attempt any theological definitions of these four central concepts. Rather, as with my patients, I will leave you with the inner traces of your early religious experience, however foreign or even abhorrent to your present consciousness they may be, and against this background I will describe each of these concepts as they emerge in my psychotherapeutic practice. I hope we will be able to note commonalities as well as differences, particularly those differences that have forced so many of us to abandon that tradition for humanism and, in more recent years, for stranger and Eastern traditions.

Let us begin with God.

What, or who, then, is God in psychotherapy? On the surface—if you listen to the patient—God is the savior. He is Godot, for whom the patient waits and who will make everything all right or at least will enable the patient to do what he has to do in order to be well. But he, God, is always coming, never there, always just around the corner or arriving on the next train. And the patient hates him for it. So God becomes "they"—the afflictor and tormentor. He without whom the patient would be fine. He is a God-Devil. You can if you wish simplify this into parental ambivalence, but the feeling goes beyond transference. God has immediate existential presence.

On the surface, to the therapist, God is the magician—the Magus, the miracle worker, often perceived by the therapist as *time* or *process*. If neither time nor process brings the miracle, he may call on the pope who dispenses sacraments—called drugs—and who, when necessary, provides sanctuary—called a hospital—for exorcism. But, on the surface, if you just listen to the words, all this is God, the God in psychotherapy.

But beneath the words, God in psychotherapy is an unending feeling in both therapist and patient. As a feeling he is no longer the savior, the protector, the refuge, the afflictor, or the tormentor. He is not the significant *other*, responsible for both my well-being and my ill-being. *He is the possible me.* And this *growth feeling*—an unending premonition of creation—is the most profound commonality linking the therapist and patient in their spiritual adventure. When feeling contact with it is lost in either one, the adventure stops, and it becomes a time of reconnoitering, of reassuring. The search ceases.

What more concretely is the possible me? To begin with it is not the *probable me*. It is not what I *could* be so much as it is what I *would* be if only the circumstances were right and I had an eternity of time. The probable me is realizable. The possible me is not realizable. Yet, paradoxically, if I merely struggle for the probable me, I tend to remain the same—with only the illusion of change. This is a common experience in psychotherapy. However, if I struggle to attain the unrealizable *possible me* I in fact gradually approximate the probable me. As the probable me, I am always in relationship. As the possible me (God), I would transform relationship, in the sense that others would be me without in the least detracting from me.

To retreat to humanistic and existential language: the *probable me* is becoming, and the *possible me* is being. Becoming is self-actualization; being is the self fully actualized. I can be more as a person only if I feel there is more to be as a person. But—and this is important—I have to believe deeply that I can be fully actualized. To put it in theological terms, to become more of a person I have to be convinced that I can become God, without becoming either angry or cynical because I never do. And I never do; and I never will, because the biological terminus of my becoming is death (unless I believe in life after death, an idea that has no consequence to me as a participant in psychotherapy). God then is not process but what motivates process.

There are two other tangible aspects of psychotherapy that could be related to God. I am convinced that one of the most fundamental aims of psychotherapy is to relieve the patient of his paranoia, to exorcise the devil. It involves the tedious task of making the patient feel genuinely that he is totally and fully responsible for everything that happens to him. No one has done anything to him—he has fully participated in everything that has happened to him. He has gotten what he wanted. In fact if he really wishes to know what it is he genuinely wants, he has only to look at what he has gotten. In that sense he is omnipotent—he totally and precisely orders his own life. *In that sense he is God*, albeit a bumbling God and a God who disavows responsibility. When and if he accepts this responsibility for self, he moves closer to the *possible me*.

Finally and briefly, I sense God in psychotherapy at those unpredictable moments in the relationship when the patient and I are fully related—usually nonverbally, generally through eye contact, and without conflict or intent. These moments provide each of us with the experience of the *possible me* in relationship. It happens.

Now let us turn to sin, the consequence of our fall from Godness.

I consider all my patients sinners, and I see my motivation for being a therapist, which involves my spending my days with sinners, as arising out of my desire to transcend my own sinfulness, my desire to be more beautiful. I do not think that God's intent in creation is at all ambiguous. I think, and this is admittedly presumptuous, that He or She or Them had in mind finding out whether man, were he free to, would choose to be God. And you will recall from my earlier remarks that choosing to be God is choosing to be a fully actualized person.

As I have said, a major part of my agenda in psychotherapy is bringing the patient to a feeling of full responsibility for himself. If he is blatantly self-destructive, helping him to accept responsibility for that is not too difficult a task. It becomes much more difficult, even tedious, to insist on his full responsibility for his own lack of gratification when, as he angrily says, he is married to a frigid woman. I am willing to go to ridiculous lengths with this if, for example, I insist he search out his participation in being mugged downtown by two hoodlums. I know realistically he may have been a victim, but I have yet to encounter complete innocence. Of course, I realize that this approach can be abused and misused by moral masochists and patients who are depressed, and it may even be subtly employed by a therapist to disown his own responsibility with the patient. "That's your problem" can be a sneaky response. But then devious, sick motives can easily dismantle the sturdiest of truths.

How does a psychotherapist help a patient become responsible for what has happened to him? Telling him he is irresponsible is simply another way of being without grace—or acceptance, as I will later describe it. It gets us nowhere.

Suppose he says, "Okay, I would like to become more responsible for me. But I don't honestly know how to recognize when I am being responsible and when I am avoiding that responsibility." Here we enter the second major part of my agenda in psychotherapy. Responsibility for self was the first; the second is morality, without which responsibility for self or others is ridiculous. So in their search for responsibility for self, patients begin seriously to explore their moral experience. The moral exploration is both necessary and inevitable in psychotherapy. It rapidly becomes evident that the patient has a moral code or imperative that resides outside him. It is another voice; someone other than him. Someone other than his own person says, "That is wrong or bad—you should feel ashamed or guilty about that" or, just as irrelevantly, "That is good—you should feel proud about that." The morality is external to the person and, so, dependent. The choice for the patient at that point is simply to conform or rebel. He feels bad in both circumstances. He is caught in the strange paradox of sin, for, if morality is prescribed by an outer moral authority, he does not really like himself whether he is bad or good. He becomes nothing in his moral subservience. He loses his essential humanness, just as he lost it in the Garden of Eden. And God in His infinite wisdom, deciding He had made a mistake, corrected it by allowing man to sin, and so freed him to become a moral creature. It was as if He decided there was no way to begin as a God, man had to work up to it—and the royal road to Godliness was moral choice, based concretely on man's freedom to sin. As if in reflecting, He decided that the quality of Godliness resided not so much in His goodness as in His freedom to be bad. So, capacity for sinning became an essential quality of humanness and a precondition for man's ascent to Godliness.

What then becomes the moral issue in psychotherapy? If the patient abandons his dependent morality—the someone outside him who dictates right and wrong—what is there left? The answer is, he is left with the labor of developing an *inner* morality, or in Carl Rogers's words, a sensitivity to his own congruence, his sense of wholeness as a person. The patient's sense of goodness or badness is to arise out of his particular and concrete experience of being at one with himself in all of his behavior. If he lives his life congruently, he likes himself, if he does not live this way, he dislikes himself. As this sensitivity develops, as the patient learns to pay passionate attention to himself rather than to others, his inner morality becomes a horrendous taskmaster. Raised a Catholic, with its demanding moral imperatives, I can tell you that these moral demands are candy-assed compared to the pain and distress I have felt when I have violated my inner sense of wholeness. I can tolerate another's disdain much more easily than I can disdain of myself. So I have come to distinguish sin from evil. Sin has to do with violating others' standards, evil has to do with violating my own person. And often I find I have to sin to avoid being evil. Above all else I have to avoid being evil. Thus, we search for the God in us and find sin; but, it is mostly evil that exhausts our beauty, and so we pray for grace to enable us to renew the search.

What is grace? I can speak of this with much feeling since my lack of it marred my beginning years as a psychotherapist with much pain. I was trained in the psychoanalytical practice. As a young analytical therapist, I felt confident of my assessments of what was wrong with my patients; I could see clearly what the problems were. I knew how they had come to be sick and the specific ways they were sick. Furthermore, I was probably right. They were sick in just those ways I thought them sick. My analytical training was more than adequate to enable me to identify their problems correctly. Once recognizing their sickness, I then moved to the problem of their rehabilitation. I knew what deficiencies had to be corrected and generally how to go about correcting them. So, reasonably, I informed my patients of their problems and expeditiously proceeded to the business of change. I knew what was wrong and what to do to change it. So I went about it.

The problem was that no one changed. They stubbornly hung on to their sicknesses, and I, equally stubbornly, hung on to my clarity about what had to be done to change that sickness. Something had to give, and after three or four years of failure, I was at least reasonable enough to know that it was I who had to change. How?

I struggled with this for years. What was wrong? I had competently identified their problems and just as competently described to them what changes had to take place and how I could facilitate these changes. Why were my patients so stubborn and recalcitrant to my competent ministry? My first clue was completely subjective. I felt proud of my patients for their stubborn refusal to change. They were right. Whatever human dignity is, my patients were more in touch with it than I was. In their stubborn refusal to change they seemed more impressively human than I, the competent and reasonable minister. Just as the horrible alcoholic husband feels more human to me than the righteous reasonable wife.

What was missing in me? It finally dawned on me that I was being in my benevolent way just another replica of my patients' parents, however malevolent they may have been. My loving benevolence could not significantly make up for the startling fact that I and their parents were identical in our relationship to them. None of us had ever accepted them as they were. We all knew what was wrong with them—the parents perhaps incorrectly and I probably correctly—and we all surely communicated to them a sense of sin and deficiency. The parents and I knew exactly what had to be done to make them good and acceptable people. Even though I was probably more reasonable than the parents, emotionally I was indistinguishable from them. It's amazing that my patients didn't shoot me.

I came then to the most significant discovery I have come to in thirty years of psychotherapy. Before you can help anyone be different, you have to accept them as they are. This is their initial experience of total acceptance, of total positive unconditional regard. Unless this occurs, nothing eventuates in therapy. This means loving—enjoying—being with them as they are, without any insistence they have to be different for you to love them. My initial reaction to this was that I could attitudinally become an accepting person and this would be sufficient. This was more philosophical than real. I soon found that the problem of acceptance was an unending problem. It had to be met as a serious relational problem in every new therapeutic relationship. And it takes time and effort in each instance. Some I cannot accept even after months. And I cannot help them. Others I can accept—it may take weeks or months—and I can help. But it is my first order of business in therapy. This acceptance of another is what I mean by grace. It is total acceptance of the others as they are with all their beauty and all their crap, without any hidden intent in such acceptance. "I love you" is graceful. And it is real, not sentimental.

Finding grace, we are then available for salvation, at first blush a rapid escalation to a guaranteed eternal Godness, but on closer examination probably the most mystical of our sacred concepts.

As a psychotherapist I think first of "savior," then I think of *salve*—the warm psychological ointment of reassurance. As long as I am the savior-therapist, I will have people coming to me to be saved. Fortunately, I am usually a failure as a savior. Patients can learn and grow from that failure. But sometimes I do save them; sometimes I am a "successful" savior. And like the revived Christian, the patient experiences a few weeks of infused pseudo-spiritual exuberance and then crashes, deciding correctly that the psychological-salvation business has limited value. It is the history of the weekend encounter. Importantly, it doesn't keep them from coming back to get saved and crash again. It sort of keeps putting God in his place. A charismatic phony like our revered parents.

But make no mistake. Patients, with few exceptions, come to

therapy to be saved. It is their initial verbal presentation. And as you would suspect, they come to be saved from something or someone—wife, husband, past, society, depression, anxiety, fate, other people, the Communists, the past, the future— saved from the enemy, something or someone other than self. Under these circumstances the only immediate danger is that they may have made an appointment with a loving salvationist.

Be they fortunate enough not to run into a loving salvationist, their initial need to be saved from the enemy moves to a deeper and more meaningful search for salvation. It moves to redemption. Redemption is more meaningful than revival. They ask to be *forgiven,* which implies that they have recognized their evil. But not completely. If you listen to them carefully, they are not yet really contrite but are actually negotiating with God. The process in therapy is not at all unlike the typical course of therapy for couples. The participants begin with months of accusing each other (the enemy theme), then move to the contrite period where each accepts his or her own faults, but, and this is a prohibitive "but," each insists that the spouse do likewise and also confess his or her contrition in the marriage. They then reasonably say to each other (argue) that if you are willing to change, I will change with you. This I call "marital negotiations."

Individual patients do this as well, except their negotiations are with God, or the therapist, or their introjects, or with their unconscious imperatives. But it is still negotiation. And negotiation with God is the hallmark of all redemptorists. If at this point they are unlucky enough to be dealing with a loving redemptorist therapist, they will settle for an adjusted impasse in their lives, or their marriages, and become what I call the adjusted ones. On the other hand, if they are once again fortunate, and are not dealing with a loving redemptorist, they may move to a still deeper experience of salvation. Loving redemptorists, by the way, have a tendency to retreat to the use of tranquilizers to redeem.

With couples, if the negotiations fail or become interminable, occasionally they move to a different relationship—a nondependent decision to make the marriage work whatever the partner does or doesn't do. I am in this marriage, it is important to me, I accept total responsibility for my experience in it, and I am going to risk simply being me, regardless of how you respond or fail to respond. Suddenly you are experiencing salvation in its most profound sense—death and resurrection. Death is nondependent being: being out of self without fear of, or concern with, possible responses from others. The deepest risk possible. To be yourself out of yourself without the unending monitoring of the possible acceptance or rejection by others. The risk of total aloneness, the risk of isolation, the risk of no community—in short, the risk of separation, of psychosis, of death. Separation and psychosis like the lonely craziness of Jesus in the desert or even in Gethsemane. Risking even more the lonely death on the cross, despised and abandoned by all. But passionately and heroically being your own person, as was Jesus. Total surrender of your dependent self. And out of that surrender, that death, that total personal being commonly called psychosis—what? Possibly, a rebirth of self. Possibly. But the risk (as described unendingly by those who never descend from the cross, the schizophrenics) is the death of both the lover and the loved. And salvation becomes possible rebirth—resurrection—rising again to assume equality with both Father and Holy Ghost (or "mother," in my terms). One becomes a fully actualized human being.

I hope you have compared these Christian concepts as they emerged in the process of my experiences in psychotherapy with the ideas of God, sin, grace, and salvation as you remember them out of the depths of your early religious engrams. If you are like me, they bear little resemblance. I also feel a resentful sadness that had I had the opportunity of immersing myself in the original Christian traditions prior to their demystification by the doctrinaire churches, Eastern traditions might not seem presently so different and attractive.

Putting such sacred nostalgia aside, however, in actual experience with my patients these sacred traditions offer little facilitation to personal search and growth. To retreat to my earlier language, they appear instead to have been massively integrated into the resistance systems of patients, either consciously or preconsciously.

Why? Are the Judaeo-Christian traditions insufficient, or even unsuitable to undergird and synergize the psychotherapeutic exploration of the human spirit? I suspect that the answer is yes, particularly as regards the correctional mainstream of that sacred tradition.

I offer two general historical explanations for this insufficiency. The first is familiar to most of you. In its beginnings the Christian movement arose as an effort to substitute love for the Judaic law as the basis for human relationships. It never quite succeeded, and because of its continued subservience to The Law, which was imposed on the person rather than emerging from the person loving, it of necessity retained an absentee, all-powerful God. Some encouragement can be taken from the splitting of Jehovah into at least three persons. It represented a significant step in the democratization of Godness, more significant than the anthropomorphizing of Godness by the Greeks. Of the three persons, the Holy Ghost offered the greatest potential as an aspect of Western tradition that might have been, and might still be, available to those struggling to evoke the human spirit or soul.

Then why has that tradition retreated and been constricted rather than grown in its obvious potential universality, modifying other traditions and being modified by others, ultimately to merge with all sacred traditions? Why the provinciality of all sacred traditions, not too unlike that of psychotherapies? I believe both are captured by their cultures, which is quite different from being assimilated by them. Capture implies stultification, whereas assimilation is a process of making something one's own and being led by it. Consequently, traditions from other cultures, even though they may be

44

captives there, represent for us an exciting reprieve from our own cultural imprisonment. For this reason the Eastern sacred traditions excite and attract those of us committed to the evolution of the human spirit. I could elaborate on the specific ways in which those other traditions would supplement our struggle with our affective concepts of God, sin, grace, and salvation in just those aspects that in the Christian tradition imprison us: the God in us, the participatory experience in the whole universe, the importance of responsibility for self, the beauty of surrender of self, the inner search, the grandness of the ordinary, and the importance of personal evil as contrasted with sin. But these are matters for another time. My advice to you then is to choose your guide carefully, whether spiritual or secular. Avoid prisoners as well as prison guards, the conforming as well as the rebellious, and seek out a gentle person who is never content to be content.

# Thomas Malone: *Questions*

*Question:* How does the feeling of acceptance first begin to show itself?

*Dr. Malone:* I don't know whether I've made it clear enough how concrete a thing this acceptance of the other is. It is not merely attitudinal. The problem with so many people is that they form an image of themselves as an accepting person, and they believe this is a valid and sufficient basis for acceptance in any particular relationship; it is *not*. In my own case, the primary thing I'm usually aware of is my *non*acceptance. And I mean even now, after thirty years as a therapist. When I see a new patient for the first time, my initial experience is almost always an awareness of *non*acceptance. And in each case this becomes a struggle for me, an internal struggle. Often I'll stay with those areas of the relationship where I feel nonaccepting. And after five or ten interviews the patient will know that this whole issue of acceptance is what is at stake for both of us, that it is a reciprocal demand and involves a concrete existential act.

Perhaps *then* the first feeling of acceptance can appear, and I wish I could say that it always takes place in terms of the eye contact that I've mentioned. That, however, is a very rare experience for me; in thirty years of therapy I don't think it has happened more than ten times. It is almost an ecstatic experience; and I'm not talking about that. So, I don't really know how to answer your question. I can scan my list of appointments at eight o'clock in the morning and I could more or less titrate for you my struggle with acceptance in terms of my initial response to my schedule. I don't even have to know the names of the specific patients. So, it's a very subjective thing, depending on many factors and forces in the relationship. Somehow, the communication system seems to change.

One of the best examples I can give you is of a rear admiral who was my patient for some time. He was one of the most compulsive, driven, migrainous, homicidal people I've ever seen. I really worked with this gentleman, and I never got anywhere. Then one day my titration of acceptance must have been enormous, because it was a tremendous struggle even to walk into the room with him. As I sat down (and I don't know why—probably just because I was feeling hopeless), I said to this rear admiral, "Do you happen to know anything about boats?"

And he started talking about boats and never stopped. For months he talked about boats and nothing else, and miraculous transformations began to occur in both him *and* me. Because I wasn't just sitting there listening; I knew what he was talking about and it had nothing to do with whether I knew anything about boats, which I do not. And that man did very well. Now what is there in this tiny experience? I can't say, exactly, but an acceptance took place in me; out of despair, acceptance appeared.

Another example is a sixty-three-year-old schoolteacher who had seven sisters. She had never been married, and none of her sisters had ever been married either. All she wanted to do was tell me about what went on between her and her seven sisters. And this she did, unendingly. And so, one day I said to her, "Martha, I can generally find one thing about a human being that I really can turn on to and really enjoy. But so help me God, I've been listening to you for six months and you're the first person in all my six years of practice that I can't find a single thing with." Well, she started to cry, and I thought I'd really hurt her feelings, but that wasn't it at all. She was actually crying out of joy, and she was crying out of joy because—as she told me later—that was the first time in her life that she had ever been the *only* person!

Well, I've written articles and a book about what happens in psychotherapy, and I've drawn pictures and outlined ten phases of what people go through—and all that is probably good. But what we all need to do is to listen to therapists when they're being really honest about what happens in therapy. Some of you may know about Robert Browning's response to Elizabeth Barrett Browning when she was reading one of his poems and said, "Robert, I've been reading this and I don't understand what you're saying here." And he said something like, "Well, it's no problem, let me read it." So he read it, and then he paced up and down a while, and then he stopped and said, "Elizabeth, when I wrote this only God and I knew what it meant. And now, only God knows." And now, when I think about all the expositions and explanations in my book, *The Roots of Psychotherapy*, about all I can say is, "My God!"

*Question:* I'd like to ask you about spiritual tradition from a slightly different angle. You've spoken about the way a religious tradition affects a psychiatric patient, but what about the way it affects the psychiatrist? I was thinking about this because I seem to have read somewhere that the number of psychiatrists and psychotherapists who commit suicide each year is greater than in any other profession. My question is: what is the relevance of sacred tradition to *you* as a therapist? How does it *touch* you?

*Answer:* In the sense that I've described it in this talk, it touches me all the time. You know, I am a priest; I'm clear about that, although it has taken me a long time to be able to say that. And I say it as someone who took a Ph.D. in clinical psychology back when most of the courses were in experimental psychology and statistics, and who went through medical school and then wrote a book that was supposed to be a definitive analysis of everything that happens empirically in psychotherapy.

Consciously, explicitly, on the level of words, sacred tradition means little to me. But affectively it is probably the most significant thing about my character and is therefore probably the most significant part of my relationship with patients. In terms of your remark about suicide, I think that without it, whatever "it" is, I would have blown my brains out years ago.

Not out of any despair with the world, but if I had not experienced what I've been talking about here, I don't think I could have stood the pain of nongrowing in me. I don't think I could have stood it.

Well, maybe I wouldn't have blown my brains out; I might have, well, perhaps I might have become a gynecologist and made a lot of money.

*Question:* You said that you've seen many people who've gotten involved in some spiritual tradition and integrated it into their defense structure, and that it therefore became a barrier to their growth instead of a liberating influence. Could you say more about that?

*Answer:* I don't think I was being as profound as you're suggesting. What I'm saying is that there are many people who come to see me who in words and in more than words use their Christian background as a kind of resistance to growth. Now, there are some exceptions to that; there's a possibility that some of the charismatic Christians I've seen in therapy may be different. I'll withhold judgment on that. But of course it is not just the words I'm talking about. It is the substructure of the words, the way that both the universe and their place in it are formulated in their preconscious mind. *That's* their resistance. You can literally see them come up to the edge of that, and they'll stop and almost shake before they'll go past it. This is very, very clear to me with my compulsive patients; because I consider compulsive defense structures as basically an expression of the Protestant ethic.

*Question:* Have you had any patients who've gone into the Eastern religions? And have they exhibited the same kind of problem?

*Answer:* I haven't had any patients who've gone into the Eastern traditions in the sense that you're asking about—that is, in a full, experiential way. Most of the people I see who are into Oriental religions relate to them more in terms of reading books; it doesn't cut into their character, their affect. So, I don't think I've had a single professional experience with a person who is genuinely into another tradition. The closest I can come is a Jehovah's Witness whom I am presently seeing. I don't know if any of you know much about them, but they are very, very different. And in terms of your question, that person is the only one about whom I would say that her religious tradition does *not* interfere with the expansion of her own humanness—which puzzles me, but it's a fact.

*Question:* Does this inner expansion, this search, ever end, or can it go on indefinitely?

*Answer:* I don't know. Long ago I turned over to my patients the problem of ending therapy. Before that, however, I used to think I knew all about facilitating the termination of therapy; it was a definite part of our training. Preparing them for the termination was supposed to be a process that started very early. But I got into all kinds of trouble with that because the more I consciously worked to help patients end the therapy, the more they hung on. And when one of them came in and said something like, "You know, Tom, I feel that there's not much reason for me to be seeing you twice a week. Why don't I just see you twice a month?" I'd say, "Fine, I think you're doing great; that's wonderful." And then there'd be the pregnant pause and the next thing I know they're making three appointments a week.

For years that was my usual experience, and, learning a little more about how human beings work, I started following my affect, my feeling. If I didn't like the person—which if I'd seen them that long was unlikely, since they wouldn't have stayed around—but if I didn't like them I wouldn't say much of anything. If I did like them, and I usually did, I would tell them I had no intention whatever of "facilitating the termination," that we'd finally gotten to the point where we could talk, explore, and be with each other, that it was creative for me and a tremendous experience, and if they thought I was going to empty a slot in my schedule that I would have to fill with an absolute stranger whom I'd have to struggle with for two years, and if they thought I was going to help them do that to me, then they must believe I'm sicker than I am. And they'd laugh, and then—they'd leave.

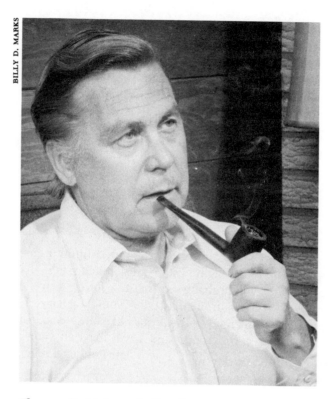

*Thomas P. Malone, M.D., Ph.D.,* is director of the Atlanta Psychiatric Clinic, P.A. and Center for Personal Growth. He is coauthor of *The Roots of Psychotherapy* and *The Psychotherapy of Chronic Schizophrenia.*

# MAN'S EVER NEW AND ETERNAL CHALLENGE

## Michel de Salzmann

First of all I wish to thank you for the opportunity I am given to speak with you tonight. But I must quickly add that the pleasure, if any, will probably be "hard"—for me as well as for you—since I am far from mastering your language. I have accepted the challenge to speak just like this—nonacademically but rather improvising—and I will need all your indulgence for the maltreatment I will inevitably give to your language.

We have, all of us, something in common—together with the fact that we just exist now: it is that to everyone present here, whether he recognizes it or not, the most important thing, the thing that really matters to him, is *himself.* I am not referring now to some specific ego features such as selfishness, self-love, or self-importance, but to something very simple, factual, quite unavoidable. Am I not extremely important since everything that exists, exists because I am? And if I think the opposite, is it not again I who think it? Everything passes through me. I am the only one who can experience or live my life. It is not a secondhand life, although unfortunately most of the time we seem to forget that.

This fact brings us immediately to the most difficult question. What is myself?

Let us try to consider that, avoiding as far as possible our "ready-made" patterns of thought. We are of course immediately tempted to refer to a philosophical point of view, or to recall the Buddhist or Hindu conception of the self, or to approach the problem in terms of depth psychology, behaviorism, or any other of our personal "idiosyncrasies." Let us try to face the question in a more provocative way, I would say in a naïve way. So I come back to myself. What is it? Do I have anything of my own?

My life? I may say, in a way it was given to me. I have done nothing for that. It is now given to me as an existential fact. I can become aware of it. It operates through my body.

This body given to me works by itself according to definite laws. It is the site of myriads of processes and of constant exchanges with the outer world. Various determining influences have given it its peculiarities: race, heredity, climate, food; and also more distant influences: astrological, cosmic, etc., of which we know very little. Anyhow, it works, and most of the time I am unconscious of it. It is like an animal. An animal in itself is a great thing, as the etymology reminds us: "anima," like "spiritus," refers to the breath, to the mysterious "animation" of the body. Thus animated, the body goes and comes, eats, sleeps, evacuates, has sex affairs and sometimes calls on me to be recognized, to be taken care of; but it usually works as well without me. In the best moments of awareness it appears to me as an integrated part of a greater whole, from which it is inseparable. Made of matter, my body obeys the causality of what we call the physical world.

Now there is another, greater whole of which I am a part, to which I belong, in which I bathe. That is culture or society. I may sometimes realize that everything I have, all my thoughts, my words, all my feelings, my body's learned ways of behavior—all the contents as well as most of the dynamics of what is called my psychological life—have been "inputted" into me.

My only originality seems to lie in the way it is put together. Everyone has a style, some characteristic habits and associations; but so it is in a computer also. The way all this has been put together has merely happened. It came about through contingency—through accidental events—and developed quite unconsciously. My computer deals with new inputs according to its own conditioned program. Nothing completely new can ever come out of it. None of us, for instance, would be able to draw an entirely new animal. Known elements or features would inevitably be made use of. I may say, roughly, and provocatively, that everything, including my character and equipment, has been given to me. My psychic life, even though it obeys the causality of intentionality, is also given to me and is basically conditioned or motivated by its cultural world.

At least something seems to remain undoubtedly my own, something that gives me the sense of my identity: I, myself, the one who pretends to be aware of all that. But here again, is it not one of those deeply rooted assumptions that we never put into question? Our "ego" actually turns out to be just as much of a gift, maybe a poisonous gift, but nevertheless a grand gift from our culture.

We are not just simply born into human existence. As existentialists would say: human existence is initially ego-consciousness. And this only appears in a child born and reared in a human society, usually after the age of two, when the neurological system has completely matured. Ego-consciousness appears then, altogether, as affirmation of oneself as I-ego; as discrimination of oneself from what is not I—the other; and as a fact presented to oneself and recognized by the ego. Immediately dissociation arises in the ego: the ego in ego-consciousness being simultaneously ego as subject and ego as object. In spite of all its dramatic attempts to escape this conditioned subjectivity, the ego seems never able to be a subject without an object . . . unless, with some help, it can go down to the very root of its fundamental contradiction.

Should I conclude that I am just a specific conjunction of

outer influences, a sort of metabolic link within the cosmos? Something remains evidently irreducible to such a perspective. However deeply I realize that what I am is altogether "imported," conditioned, and divided, I still believe in a mysterious and compelling vocation: that of being myself. Like Isis desperately trying to gather together the dispersed members of Osiris, the ego is ever in quest of a unified, meaningful identity.

In fact with ego-consciousness and its provocative ambiguity there has been awakened in us a strange and immediate sense of responsibility. This brings me much nearer to what I can recognize as my own. Especially if I recall that to be responsible means properly to respond, to answer. All I can possibly do, as a matter of fact all I am doing, is responding, responding to my existence. What really defines and shows us a man is his response. If there is for me the slightest possible choice in the midst of operating laws, whether from hazard or necessity, is it not in the way I respond—that is, in the quality of my participation in all that is given to me through the immediate experience of my life?

Let us be clear that my genuine responsiveness is not to be found in any of the formal responses that my programed computer never fails to produce. It has to be sought beyond that. It is an intentional act of knowing, which has a singular capacity for freedom since it can exist beyond my "formal" conditioning. This primary, free response is my attention. My attention is my own and fundamental answer to my existence. It is both my response and what I can be responsible for. An opening as well as an engagement, it is my becoming present to what is, it is *hic et nunc* my participating in the actuality of being. Arising as a basic act of knowing through actual being, my attention is simultaneously awakening to myself and to the world. All the rest, I mean all the other responses which are formal, all my acting out, all my outward manifestations proceed, so to say, by themselves, depending in their quality on the quality of my attention.

The idea of quality of attention is not familiar to us, nor is the idea of different possible levels of attention. But this would need an elaboration we cannot make here. Let us just say that our attention is much more than we generally think. It is much more than a simple mental or cerebral mechanism. It concerns our whole being. If its potentialities are far from being fully actualized in our usual life, maybe it is precisely because it is not recognized as a multidimensional keyboard and as the unifying principle of our being.

Paradoxically this basic act of knowing, which is attention, is only actualized when we don't know—that is, when there is a question. Its level and, so to say, its degree of "totalization" are proportional to our questioning. You have surely noticed that when a question is vital—when it takes us in the guts, as you say—it suspends all unnecessary movements, emotional and physical as well as mental. It clears the way for real awareness and sensitivity, which are components of my total power of attention. It is only between my not knowing and my urge to know that I find myself present, mobilized, open, new—that is to say, attentive.

Attention in its active form is therefore inseparable from interrogation; it is essentially, in its purity, an act of questioning. This act is the privilege of our human existence. An animal contents itself with being. The responsibility of man is to question himself on the meaning of his being.

In our society, mainly concerned with production and efficiency, the drama is that our capacity for questioning, still so vivid in early childhood, is very quickly eradicated or pushed aside for the benefit of our capacity for answering. When a child has a real question, most of the time he is immediately given a stupid answer. In the best cases the educator goes to the dictionary to be sure his answer is accurate. But anyhow unconsciously, if not proudly, he closes the question. From school to the end of our life it is always necessary to answer. We are compelled to learn how to answer. If we don't know how to answer, we are just no good. So little by little we become some kind of model machine able-to-answer-to-all-situations with all the necessary blindness as regards its own contradictions. That kind of answering, whose degree of sophistication may sometimes hide from us its conditioned character, is required by our life. But under its dominating necessity, is it possible to keep alive in ourselves our most authentic and precious capacity, which is questioning?

This is the whole problem confronting us, actually. But are we strong enough, free enough, concerned enough to really question ourselves while answering? The challenge is just as difficult as facing a Zen koan. While playing our part, while being engaged without cheating in the situation that calls us, can we at the same time neither affirm nor deny, neither resist nor follow, assume that we neither know nor don't know, that we are able or unable? Can we be acutely present to what is, without judgment or indifference, without any solution or escape? It would mean being aware on all fronts, renouncing the known for the unknown, withstanding the inevitable principle of repetition, staying still within our movement.

Total questioning in our living is the key to being, but whoever ventures unprepared into the experience will meet a wall of resistance in himself, if not simply fear that he is stupid, incapable, and so on. Only exceptionally motivated searchers will take the risk and leave room for questioning—and get beyond the phantasms of insecurity. Most of us are so busy with successful answering and so identified with our own image that we need severe shocks such as death, suffering, illness, deep frustration, or "supergratification" to awaken to the question.

The question is here, waiting for us, following us everywhere, since we ourselves are that very question. I have started with it, asking, "What am I?" but this approach has kept me an outsider, a mere on-looker of myself. When born in the mind, the question calls forth an answer through the mind and keeps me divided under my compulsion for explanation and for power over my object world. Understanding needs more. It needs experiencing—that is, to be put to the test and to pass through. I have to engage myself, to respond totally in the act of knowing myself. Arising from being, the question finds an answer through being. Our question has thus shifted from a ratiocentric point of view to an ontocentric point of view and has become "Who am I?"

Behind the misleading screen of all the other questions it is the question of each man in his human existence. It is his first and last question. It is today as it was centuries ago. Throughout human history, dim, bright, or enlightening lights have repeatedly reactivated that question. It is the axis around which moves in a spiral the eternal revolution of human culture.


I have tried to convey in this sequential approach that all human "problematic" derives from a fundamental alienation, arising with ego-consciousness, which naturally and necessarily loads every human being with the responsibility to question and find his own identity, his real meaning, his freedom. The symptomatic evidence of the problem, behind its polymorphic expression, is human suffering and consequently the need for help, for an answer. Psychotherapy and traditional spiritual teachings have themselves originated from the need to resolve this alienation, to answer our central existential question, "Who am I?" Considering them against the background of this question referring to being is not a mere tautology. It provides a relativistic perspective which not only contains them both but includes all of us. And furthermore, it will help to clarify why, although they answer the same need, I consider they should not be confused, especially if we realize they are operating on two different levels.

It must first be clear that our present theme leaves almost entirely aside the major part of the psychiatric field. Alteration of ego-consciousness, abortive, retarded, deteriorated, or regressed, is not within our consideration here. Our theme refers to a relatively sound ego, which is able to see, and to recognize as its own, its problems, its contradictions, its conflicts, or its limitations—an ego whose suffering gives rise to a conscious wish to clarify and handle its situation and which actively seeks help either in psychotherapy or in spiritual guidance. But even though limited to the almost standard situation, the problem still involves, in the background, the necessity of a consistent psychopathological doctrine, which alone can dissipate the confusion about the difficult question of the limits of psychiatry.

It is also clear that I cannot speak in the name of either psychotherapy or spiritual teachings as such. I certainly would be at a loss if I would even try to take a thorough census of all their manifestations. But on the other hand, I am not considering them as an outsider. For a good many years I have personally studied, experienced, worked along specific lines in both fields, and through that engagement I have tried to understand many other lines as well as I could. Both realms are definitely of great concern to me.

Generally speaking I would call them both schools of self knowledge. Their kind of knowledge has unusual practical implications. It has to be embodied. Its double exigency is to be in order to know what one is and to know in order to be what one knows.

By both schools we are told that we live in ignorance of ourselves, separated from ourselves, that we have to discover and reunify ourselves in order to be or become what we really are. For both of them the way is consciousness. In their most authentic or genuine form, they support us in the difficult way to pure attention, where our existential duality may be experienced and perhaps even resolved. All their concepts, protocols, rituals, techniques, and severe disciplines serve as necessary but provisional media or supports for the actualization of the potentialities of being, through self-consciousness.

When these schools degenerate, the basic and practical striving for consciousness disappears, giving way to uncontrolled released forces, to magical or wishful thinking, to suggestion, self-securization, imitation, and blind repetition. Instead of conveying an awakening influence, their knowledge becomes either dead or dangerous, fostering conventional, normative, institutionalizing patterns or even delirious "trips" or hysteria.

We have to admit, from a practical point of view, that teachings become what men make of them; they are what the men are who convey them. I only wish to refer to what seems serious to me: namely, the transmission of knowledge, and guided experience, in which the guides honestly know what they are doing and know their own limitations, know precisely what they are working on, the ways and means, the necessary conditions and indications, the objective results, and are able to adjust general principles to individual situations.

I certainly think that serious engagement in either psychotherapy or spiritual paths may equally bring at least a taste of openness, of self-awareness, of self-transcendence and inner harmony. Nevertheless, however difficult it may be to trace it, a line (or, better, a border of transition) exists, and must exist, that separates the therapeutic process from an authentic spiritual work or transformation—a line that separates the pathological condition from higher levels in human existence. In fact, it is only if their demarcation is looked upon as separating different levels of being, and not merely different fields of operation, that these human experiences can be comprehended in both their underlying similarity and their outstanding difference.

This requires that we consider being from a genetic or evolutionary perspective, in which there recurs, on each level, the central problem of freedom and, correlatively, of alienation.

Considered in terms of the conditions of our culture, the ego in ego-consciousness, through the developmental phases that constitute the progressive integration of its object world, organizes itself into a subject that is able to relate freely to its world, inner and outer, and to act under the control of its reason. Maturity in our human existence is thus not a mere social adjustment or normalization but the attaining of free will, of autonomy, by which the ego is and feels free (although simultaneously responsible) for its choices, its ends, its proximate destiny.

The loss or nonattainment of "free responsibility"—or in other words, regression or fixation to lower organizations of being, where the ego is more or less entirely bound to its phantasms—is psychopathology. "Pathology of freedom" of the ego as subject, as a person, is the legitimate and traditional field of psychiatry and, by extension, of psychotherapy. It delimits the alienation of some men, as set apart from all the others by mental illness.

It seems impossible to deny (and nobody does so convincingly) the reality of madness, of pathological alienation. Yet this is what an exclusive adherence to sociopsychogenetic conceptions of mental disease may lead to. Extending the field of psychopathology to the whole system of relations within the family and society, although in many respects justified, leads, when too radical, to absurd doctrinal positions. In its extremism, antipsychiatry negates the psychiatrist and mental illness together, both being considered artificial expressions of a sick society. Of course, it is just as easy for some theorists in psychiatry to point out all the sophisms included in such conceptions. If the mad are not different from all people, it follows that all people are mad, which is the same as saying that nobody is mad. Burning the psychiatrist in the illusory hope of making a guru out of his ashes is confusing the phenomenon of madness with that of general alienation, the alienation common to all men. It is to confuse the different levels of organization of being and to reduce man to his cultural dimension alone. But, so as not to discard here what may be valuable in these trends of thought, let us agree with Leibniz that the inevitable drama of any ideology is that "it is true in what it affirms and false in what it negates."

Without going deeper into these theoretical considerations, we will say that psychopathology, and therefore psychotherapy, loses its specificity when it confuses pathological alienation with general alienation. This confusion results from loose conceptions of mental illness, in which the necessary biological dimension is lacking, in which psychiatry is cut off from medicine, and being from its infrastructural reality and structural unity.

It seems to me that only holistic theories, such as, for instance, Henri Ey's "organo-dynamic" conception—which is in the line of neo-Jacksonism and which I find exceptionally broad and coherent—may help to elucidate the mystery of the structural gap that always exists between mental disorders (either organic or functional) and clinical symptomatology. Mental illness, according to this conception, is considered a disorganization of the psychic being which presents both a negative and a positive aspect. Negatively, it is the dissolution, destructuration, or regression into a lower level of organization of being or of consciousness. This negative aspect is the *illness,* which only a biological approach can explain. The *positive* aspect is the liberated expression of this more primitive level, in which the *person* organizes his intentionality, and which only the psychological sciences can understand.

If we neglect the negative aspect in mental illness and emphasize only the positive aspect (that of liberated pathetic human expression), we are led to the error of identifying ourselves completely with the tragedy of madness—even to the extent of extolling this pathological experience—which certainly can give rise to exceptional insights but which can never lead to an effective realization of inner growth. The absurd consequence of this natural empathy is finally to equate, as has often been done, wisdom and schizophrenia, the suprarational and the infrarational. It shows a complete misinterpretation of authentic spiritual experience, which requires, for the awakening of unactualized potentialities, the highest level of integration of the body into consciousness.

The delimitation of its own object—mental illness—appears, therefore, to be a necessary condition for individualizing psychiatry among other anthropological sciences, and especially for preventing an abusive extension of its field, the "psychiatrization" of our society—that is, making psychiatry our new religion. The frontiers of psychotherapy can only be legitimately extended, in my view, if it is redefined as an educational enterprise, a modern form of support for the aspiration and initiation toward inner growth.

It is only too evident that freedom of the ego, as previously referred to, is highly relative and conditioned, that a sensitive and responsible man is confronted with an alienation shared with others, which we will assume can only find its resolution in a higher consciousness of his being. Furthermore he is not yet an individual, in the sense that he is still divided in the dualistic structure of the ego, always returning to being a subject separated from its unfathomable object.

Psychotherapy is of inestimable value if it can foster in a man his questioning or an active reflection upon himself and help him, through various kinds of conscious experience, to explore more deeply his entire functional world and all possible influences that condition his existence. It will reach its highest standards if it develops in us a sense of solidarity toward mankind and its common alienation, if it effectively engages us to work actively with others toward resolving (through questioning together) the most central of all cultural problems.

So, if the first task of psychology is to help a person to become a "free and conscious egoist," its second task, which is more educational, would be to stimulate him to become a full member of the community, as an active promoter of its becoming.

To feel oneself at one with society and within existence means entering the field of religion. Religion is not at all a personal thing; it is a public concern. It is what binds man to his whole world. It is what all men have in common. It is, etymologically, that which relates. It really starts when "egocentrism" begins to leave room for a higher level of being, which induces a new perception of one's existence. From this point of view, we can consider that psychotherapy in many instances could serve as a valuable preparation before entering into an authentic spiritual work.

Here, then, is a fundamental difference between psychotherapy and religion. We go to psychotherapy for ourselves in order to resolve our personal problems, to be helped. It is at our disposition, and we use it for our own sake, even if we realize it can benefit others indirectly. But religion is calling us to give ourselves to it. It is not there for us, until we understand that we belong to it. We are part of a whole which needs to be acknowledged now, and as ever-present. We can be greatly helped but only if we are first willing to help. It requires us to be already mature, standing on a level on which reality is more attractive than our "ego business." Zen Buddhism has become popular in the United States, so you doubtless know the Zen story of Shen-kuang. Wishing to meet Bodhidharma, who apparently does not wish to receive him, Shen-kuang stands all night at the gate through a terrible snowstorm. In the morning Bodhidharma finds him with snow up to his knees and asks him why he came. When Shen-kuang expresses his wish to follow the way, he is answered that the way is beyond human strength and would need exceptional determination. Shen-kuang then immediately takes his sword and cuts off his left arm, which he offers to Bodhidharma.

This would be, to say the least, a rather unusual occurrence in psychotherapy. It is true nevertheless that in some schools the strength of the ego, of its motivation, may be tested through raising all kinds of formal or nonformal difficulties. But such tests usually serve to reveal how the ego deals with its desire in the context of the reality principle. In spiritual paths the problem is for the ego to be determined enough in its radical choice to undergo being sacrificed for something greater. The ego in ego-consciousness must be conveyed to its own death, so to say, thus making possible the rebirth of a real "individual" in the new condition of *self-consciousness*—this new self being described as no other, or coincident with, or a reflection of the universal SELF.

Let us now consider another aspect that differentiates spiritual research from research based on an underlying scientific attitude, and which is expressed at least in part in the distinction that is often made between explaining and understanding. Science is based on objective and object knowledge, isolating objects and explaining their manifold causal relationships. This knowledge ignores the subject, perhaps because it comes from it and so is totally identified with it. It nevertheless reinforces the subject in its entire confidence in the mind and its possibilities. It projects the searcher toward the object world, scattering him through the endless accumulation of data. We are able to integrate all that knowledge into systems but unable to integrate it into ourselves. We are so loaded with knowledge that we simply don't know what to do with it, how to handle it. Understanding, on the other hand, not only considers human existence in its intentionality or its causality in view of an end, it also involves referring the experience to oneself, integrating it into oneself, integrating it into being. Science can explain functioning but cannot explain wisdom or love. They can only be understood through being wise or loving. Thus the particularity of this latter kind of knowledge is to bring us back to ourselves. The first kind of knowledge is purely mental or rational, the other is not necessarily irrational but it requires the whole of ourselves, including thought.

There is a total misunderstanding, it seems to me, in the current attitude toward rationality. It is often the target of confused spiritualism, and inversely inner experience or religion is often considered irrational. The real power of the mind is attention. Rationality is the way our thought or our reflection proceeds.

It is not the mirror of reality but is relative to a system of reference, our logic, which changes and evolves. Our common logic, following the old principle of noncontradiction, has been superseded by logic implied in dialectical thought as developed since Hegel; it is transcended by the relativity of Einstein and completely struck down by the conceptions of present-day physicists and researchers.

In brief, rationality is a fundamental instrument but it is not our whole being, so the important thing is not rationality itself but the fact that most of the time our center of gravity is in the mind and not in our whole being. This is what is really difficult to convey when it has not been experienced thoroughly.

We must not forget that psychotherapy as a science, in spite of its spectacular transformation, remains nevertheless rooted in the nineteenth century's unconscious prejudices. The cult of scientism, with its God (scientific progress), its saint (the mind), and its credo ("what cannot be explained by science today, will be explained tomorrow or the day after tomorrow"), has left deep traces, keeping the searcher an outsider, even though idolatry of the mind and its supposed objectivity has been progressively and greatly demystified.

In my view, two of the richest and most revolutionary contributions of psychoanalysis have been its putting into question the credibility of the "conscious mind" and its inclusion of the researcher himself, as a whole, in the field of his study. Research can now open into the pathway of inner exploration, lived in as widely and deeply as possible.

But were these contributions sufficient to escape the trap of the mind?

In spite of experience that included the emotional and sensory, in spite of the pathos and authenticity of what was actually lived, were not the unconscious and its dialectic recaptured by the mind at the level of speech, since the Freudian consciousness seemed to limit itself to the dimension of words and since words themselves, in their signification and their interpretation, did not escape the jurisdiction of the conditioned ego? Words inevitably bring one back to the known instead of making it possible to emerge upon a radical

experience of the unknown. The mind wa
remain the touchstone of experience.

The need to go beyond the conditioned
rise to existential and phenomenological app
principal idea of "comprehension" (*Verst*
longer a matter of explaining but of being o
being, in seeking to participate without falling into the trap
and the prejudices of the mind.

This resolutely "naïve" step—naïve in the best sense, that of
being born with experience—was to prompt the Western
researcher to bring out again and give new meaning to a
concept that had long been stored away in a drawer: that of
consciousness.

For the past ten years a trend—as dynamic as it is
anarchic—has taken shape, looking for an ever greater exploration and expansion of this famous "consciousness." Granting
also a place of privilege to the notion of being, this trend has
naturally discovered with interest the existence of the traditional spiritual way, whose basis and preoccupation can be
defined as the realization or science of being.

No doubt this interest stems from the recognition that
authentic religion is an existential experience into higher levels of being and not regression into some kind of "pseudo-
nirvanic" self-security. Nevertheless the result of translating
into ordinary psychological terms some of the conceptions and
related techniques of the East may be just complete misunderstanding. Not only distortions but real dangers may result from
not approaching them with the appropriate keys and from
misusing them. It is evident that religious exercises are not
intended to benefit the ego but, as was said before, to serve the
opposite striving for a liberation from the ego, from a subject
centered in the mind.

Religion is a very high "university." Its knowledge embraces
everything. It includes on different levels a metaphysical,
cosmological, and psychological teaching. An appropriate
approach to the language of the sacred, in itself, would include

e study of many related "sciences," ranging from numerology to that of breathing. Religion is in fact a union, a "yoga" that takes place between two levels that are reflected in gnosis and praxis. In my view, the present attraction to Eastern ways is mainly due to the fact that praxis, the entire engagement of the body, fills a lack which is strongly felt in our Western mode of existence.

Such religion is not a mere sentimental journey. It is dealing with energy. It is a science of inner energy processes. This is why spiritual work needs special and competent guidance. It is evident, as regards practical knowledge about inner energy, that our approach to relaxation or sexuality, for instance, is extremely childish in comparison with what is known in traditional teachings.

I think that psychotherapy, in its new trends, has embarked upon a very difficult challenge—which I myself have long experienced—having to do with reconciling two aspects of human progress that at first sight appear irreconcilable: evolution of knowledge and evolution of being. And they will be irreconcilable as long as the first dominates the second.

This difficulty or apparent contradiction can be very simply illustrated.

Knowledge in psychotherapy is evolving, is in progress. A psychoanalyst, for instance, may think he is much indebted for his knowledge to Freud, but he assumes that many new discoveries have been made since then, so he can know much more than Freud did. In this perspective, mental knowledge evolves, is endlessly adding something new. Traditional knowledge seems entirely the contrary. It is eternal, it does not change. It evokes a reality that does not change but has to be recognized through a change in our being. This change takes place thanks to the help of an influence which reaches us through a spiritual linkage, an influence coming from a higher level of being. It has to be transmitted through evolved beings so that it can be alive today and still be of concern to us. It has to be spoken of rightly—which is benediction—so that it can be factually experienced, since it cannot be received in our usual state of being, that of alienation. This influence is vital to man and acts upon him. Even if he is denying it, it reminds him of the dimension of being. This is why in a traditional perspective the past is so important. It is exemplary. As a friend of mine often mentions in his lectures, the Greeks have a word, *prosten*, which means "before, in front" but designates the past; whereas the word *episten*, meaning "behind," designates the future. This reminds us that our ancestors are our "ante-cessors," or those who have been ahead of us on the way, who have already passed the "puerta del sol." They have lived what we have not yet lived, they serve as an example for us and as guides. We need their experience now that we are on the stage of life, showing by our acts what we really are, what we understand, how we exist. But this state of mind is very far from our modern way of thinking.

Let us emphasize again here, in summary, that only the dimension of being gives knowledge its different possible levels, which the mind alone cannot grasp.

Now, I think I would much prefer having questions from you. But before that I may perhaps say a few more words about the difficulty involved in deepening the act of questioning I so often referred to.

The whole problem is the passage from an ego- (or mind-centered) questioning to a self- (balanced or total) questioning. It can be considered more practically as a shift of the center of gravity of our attention from the mind to a particular center within our body. Many people today, over their cocktails, talk about the *hara*. But, as some other people say, the map is not the real territory. In fact, it is only when the "mind stops talking" that some experience of myself begins to be possible, because the center of gravity of my attention then ceases to be enmeshed unconsciously and passively in the centrifugal energy stream that invests the object. (The "object" can be also an image or abstract problem in the mind.) So my center of gravity becomes reincorporated within its only meaningful ground, in which self-consciousness has its natural roots. I mean that the field of corporeality is then reactivated or *re-membered.* Being no longer "senseless," I can now sense that my abiding-in-myself is nevertheless very threatened, very fragile; I have no balance yet, and this will be so as long as my inner energy is strongly polarized toward the mind, as long as I identify myself with this mental activity, in which I thus remain a subject alienated to an object. But if I go on wholly experiencing (as I would, for instance, during systematic relaxation), a radical change takes place when the mind gives up, sacrifices its usurped power, and yields its protective attention to the increased awakening or awareness of the body. A new balance appears in myself around the subtle sensation of an inner presence. I would call this sensation "attention of the body." I am then aware of myself as a dynamic field of forces.

Without corresponding experiencing, it is almost impossible to speak of the next step—that is, the awakening or attention of the feeling, which through a similar sacrifice brings a third dimension to my awareness: awareness of rediscovered being. Such feeling has the property of bringing a new quality of energy unifying the still "divided self."

I would say, to simplify, that each of these functional apparatuses (thought, sensation, and feeling) carries a specific energy and a specific attention or sensitivity. When mobilized together by virtue of questioning, they potentialize each other and contribute to the rare experience of being really present, aware of oneself. Everyone has tasted more or less strongly such a state of awareness in certain occasions or events of his life.

When more aware of ourselves, we are able to contain our energy and at the same time remain, so to say, open, permeable, seeing and yet not interfering in whatever has to take place in ourselves. This is already a great inner change. But even more is needed. I would like to convey what I mean through an image.

Total awareness means being present to everything within ourselves at the same time. Containing everything equally and at the same time would be idealistically possible within a sphere or circle. Well, to make a circle a center is needed. The real difficulty of finding a center in ourselves is due to movement, because everything moves. It moves from top to bottom—it is life. To resist life is nonadjustment. But there is a way, I think, to accept the movement of life and yet not be displaced. It is possible if I experience at the same time that "I am not only that."

This occurs, in fact, when I become aware of two simultaneous movements of energy that take place within myself and which I may recognize as inherent in universal life. One is an outward movement going toward the phenomenal world either outside or inside myself, the other an inward movement going toward what we have called our inner presence, which does not change throughout the years. The first movement pertains to the uninterrupted creative process and the other is the movement of return to its source, to apparent undifferentiation, which I may also call death. The second of these movements, it seems to me, is usually not taken into account in the modern idea of consciousness. The drive for "expanding consciousness" seems too often to be a new, covert wish for the ego to expand. I think, as we are, there is nothing to expand but much to retract. We have to learn how to come back.

The question is whether we can participate consciously and simultaneously in these two currents in our daily life. If we can, maybe we can completely transform our impression of ourselves and our inner attitude toward life.

The second movement, that of death, is the more difficult for us to understand. I do not consider it at all in the sense of entropy, or as a drive toward a static state of no tension. We should understand it as the reversed dynamism of life, the ascending movement of evolution, which is necessarily contained in the whole process expressed in the concept of revolution or cycle.

I do not wish here to enter into any of the metaphysical principles of traditional teachings or the correlative findings of advanced science, since other people are doing it much better than I can. But without considering the problem of simultaneity of existence and nonexistence, of movement and nonmovement, I may just briefly touch on the idea of the universal cyclic process.

We can consider any given phenomenon as the transformation of energy within a specific cycle which itself belongs, through participation, to a cycle of greater scale, and this one in turn belongs to a still greater cycle, and so on—like the Russian dolls, if you wish. Time itself is not only linear but also an expression of the cyclic process of existence. It is relative to the scale of each particular cycle, of its whole revolution. Since universal movement never stops, time expresses itself, on each cyclic level, by rhythm. Temporality is directly expressed, for instance, in the beating of our temples, of our *temporal* vessels. The life of an organism taken as a whole represents likewise the revolution of a cycle (which is, so to say, harmoniously polyrhythmic). Whether this process lasts for a microsecond, an hour, a day, a month, a year, a hundred years, or a thousand millennia, it remains fundamentally identical to the "whole"— which is beyond temporality. We may have an extraordinary key to many questions if we consider that the entire cycle of existence of a given organism (or natural phenomenon) on one scale is contained within the cycle of a single breath (comprising expiration and inspiration) on another scale. Hindu tradition thus speaks of the breathing of Brahma as being the breathing of the whole universe, containing these two movements of involution and evolution which are taking place simultaneously and pervading all Creation.

Oneness in this dual movement is and remains the supreme challenge of life to man's questioning. Both science and religion are sacrificing to the mystery of unity in multiplicity. It engages us more than a mere theory or belief. We can be a holist or a monist. But being ONE in ourselves and in our Self is more difficult than to be a monist by thought.

Well—this awkward monologuing in English must have an end. It will be a great help if you enter the discussion. . . .

# Michel de Salzmann: *Questions*

*Question:* I was touched by something you said about the attention of the feeling. I wonder if you could say a little more about what that might mean?

*Dr. de Salzmann:* It is what is often referred to as the opening of the feeling, of the heart. But, you see, we are always speaking of these things in a conceptual way. It makes the approach nearly impossible, since this kind of experience should be dealt with in terms of energy. The opening of the feeling can only take place when one begins to understand, through experience, the necessity of a balanced state in the distribution and circulation of our inner energy. It involves a new center of gravity of attention, its withdrawal from the mind, and the revelation, here and now, through my entire body, of my existential participation in life. In that state, for instance, the act of breathing can be in itself an entirely new experience. It engenders a specific shock and mobilization of energy when I discover that "it breathes through me." And if I can let it be and am able not to interfere, not to react in any manner to it, it awakens a new kind of sensitivity. This, for instance, can open in me something quite unusual, but it comes through a special balance, I would say.

I have already spoken of something that also seems important to me. It is intensity. It is only when a man is involved beyond his limits—which are to a great extent imaginary—when he cannot make it, when he cannot take the situation, when he does not know how to face it or cope with it and feels overwhelmed by it, then, only then, is suddenly awakened a full attention of the *whole* of oneself.

Psychotherapy makes it possible to taste this to a certain extent. It is more frequently approached, I think, through the dynamics of a group experience. But usually it is not consciously brought up for its own sake and does not awaken the whole of ourselves. It is an important characteristic of a

76

genuine traditional way to know how to put someone suddenly, through a question or situation, in such suspense that he can't take it only with the mind, that it calls equally an awareness in the body and in the feeling. Like being in front of a koan. He is just there! He can't quit, he can't go forward, backward, up, or down—he can't go anywhere. To be in such a situation (which also means to accept it) brings a quality of awareness impossible to find otherwise, except in very difficult accidental situations that life provides us with. But in the latter case we are not able to appreciate our chance to be in such a situation and we are only occupied with finding a way out. Nevertheless it remains unforgettable. We realize we felt astonishingly alive, but without knowing why, so very often we try to reproduce this situation, to repeat it. But it cannot be repeated. We have to be new. And, by the way, that is not available through any drug.

*Question:* I realize that in my ordinary way I'm not balanced. I even see in a way what is typically out of balance and I wish to come into balance. It seems to me that what gets in my way is the concern, the exact experience of being out of balance, when that could be just the experience I need.

*Answer:* This is, I think, exactly the key. This is where a real need comes from. This is where our real help comes from. To be out of balance is my greatest help if I only realize it and see that "I" cannot balance myself. This egoistic wish to which I cling is just the continuation of what keeps me out of balance. It needs to be understood in a new way. "I" cannot make it myself, and as long as I stick to the wish to be balanced, the imbalance goes on. Again, only when I am overwhelmed, when I cannot face the situation, can something entirely new appear that helps me to understand what is really needed.

*Question:* What do you mean by there being two movements, in and out?

*Answer:* I think only one thing makes it possible to change our situation. It is sacrifice. But we should not take it in a sentimental way. Sacrifice means literally "to make sacred": *sacrum facere.* It is turning toward, canalizing energy toward, a new direction. It is what permits one to abandon, to free oneself from one's, identification with the outward movement. We are completely identified with the creative movement, if I may say so. The movement that goes toward multiplication of phenomena, the inevitable fruits of action. There is a terrible wastage of everything on earth in relation to that, in fact. The traditional attitude is far from our profane way of living. For instance, the simple act of eating, of taking food, would imply the effective awareness that the intake of energy is not only destined to sustain my little person; it should mainly, so to say, nourish God within me. I myself have more life only if He is more animated. This is the meaning of sacrifice. It is making alive in ourselves an inner process, which needs to be nourished as materially as any other energy process. When we are thus recalled to the evidence of this inner dimension, we cease to project completely to the outside, we cease being enslaved to what we think we are and what we think we should be, should do, and so on. You are recalled to something forgotten, and if you listen to it you may suddenly realize there is another process that might take place in you, which shifts your attention to a new center of gravity. That other process we usually ignore completely. It is quite material, not idealistic, but we have to approach that point to recognize it.

*Question:* What bases are there to study all this? I mean, you just don't know who you are. What do you study?

*Answer:* The basis is just what authentically you *need* to know. If you put the question like that, there is no real necessity. But any question can be a start as long as it is yours. If *you* have the real need to answer any of your questions, you will stop everything, you will look, inquire, investigate, you will go everywhere, and you will have help. Maybe you will realize you just can't answer this questioning once and for all. You have to serve it actively. Well, it's already a very high thing not to forget it in order not to stop its inner progress. I think it's already great. Then I would say you don't need a psychiatrist any more!

*Question:* Is fear a property of the ego-consciousness?

*Answer:* Of course in a human being fear is mainly related to the problem of the image of oneself, to the identification with this image and the phantasms of its being threatened. In animals images, memory, or associations also exist, but fear is not anticipated, it does not exist out of an immediate realistic context. There are many aspects to that question. We are governed by our associations, much more so than we think. Fear-related associations differ greatly with people. It is instructive, for instance, from a very simple practical point of view, to see these differences between us. Some people are more free or courageous with their mind. They don't fear to have some strange ideas, or even hallucinations. Some others will be more courageous as far as their body engagement is concerned but are not able to face internal conflicts. Fear is a fundamental problem. Very large. Maybe the basic fear is *not to be.* So it is only when you die, when you die to yourself, that you are delivered from fear, because then you discover the realm of being.

*Question:* I felt I needed to hear what you were saying and it moved me, it touched me. I'm very interested in the idea of death, and in our culture it's very difficult to come across situations or individuals, in a very broad sense, where death is faced, where one is somehow allowed to explore it.

*Answer:* We can only observe and know things when they happen. Now again, what seems to me practical and most important is to have a question. But the difficulty is to carry it, to carry it into real experience, because questioning is an act, it is not something of the mind. It is an act by which you become completely available. One can say that if a man were able to mobilize himself completely, totally, through his questioning who he is, he would be. The question would be resolved by his simultaneously appearing—that is, by his becoming present, by his entire self-consciousness, if you see what I mean. So, how can you, how can we, experience, and not remain in the nets of the mind, whether dogmatically or not? I think the very fact of experiencing the act of interrogation is already an answer to the question of death. It is somehow, in its essential movement, participating also in the death process.

*Question:* Could you say something about the differences between one's male and female aspects? I have found that some parts of myself are neither one nor the other, are not feminine or masculine, they're just there, not one or the other completely. And yet what I seek seems to be a property of something, I don't know, maybe male; and because I seek it I can't be it.

*Answer:* It's a very large problem, a universal problem. Would there be something male without the female? They go always together, like two complementary forces. We need the whole to understand each one in its relation to the other. You would not exist if you didn't have both already. You are a result of their action and still carry them. One can say that at every moment, on different scales, these two principles are working and meeting in you, accomplishing and renewing a never-ending creative process. In that perpetual movement death and birth coexist constantly but on many different scales. We have spoken of that. You are composed of different bodies on different scales.

In each atom, cell, organ, function, and in each individual as a whole the two principles are operating simultaneously. One is active, the other passive, relative to one another. (The principle and scale of relativity might, of course, enable us to consider each force in itself in another relational perspective.) Between them or from them something new is created, which in its turn participates and acts within the general cycle of evolution and involution.

So, you represent something as a whole. So as a whole you would like to be what? If you seek to be male, active, it will certainly operate in a way, but then maybe you will not be activated by something more active or male, which is beyond you. This may be one of the real choices we have. It is only when you are passive from a certain point of view that you receive, that you are fecundated by some spiritual force. You see, there are many ways to consider that problem. Only a perspective of relativity gives us the necessary flexibility to adjust to what is in movement, in perpetual becoming. Concepts and definitions are too static to dance with life. Only traditional or mathematical symbols show the way for that kind of thinking.

*Question:* In trying to know myself, I see that I need to study my experiences, to experience things more fully. It seems that psychotherapy allows me to have a wider range of experiences for me to know myself than is true of our traditional ways and I'm wondering why that is.

*Answer:* Only you can answer this! But this is exactly why, in my opinion, it is almost impossible to mix these two ways. Except under special conditions, it should be one after the other, or one or the other.

*Same questioner:* In the traditional ways there often seems to be a judgment that things I might think or do or feel are somehow wrong. I find this less true in relation to the psychotherapist. He seems to accept these eccentricities of mine.

*Answer:* Maybe you have to go forward until you come to a point where you will not mind yourself so much and feel much freer. I recall some good words I have read lately. Saint Augustine said, "Love God and do what you like." He didn't say, "Love what you like, that's God."

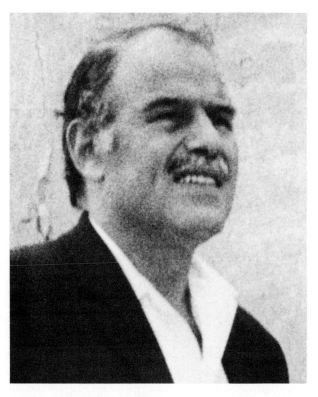

*Michel de Salzmann, M.D.*, fifty-one years old, is a French psychiatrist living in Paris. For the past twenty years, in addition to his work in individual psychotherapy, he has been leading research groups in inner growth in France, Switzerland, Holland, and occasionally in the United States. Every summer he conducts international seminars. He travels widely throughout Asia and the Middle East in order to study traditional teachings at first hand.

# TIBETAN BUDDHISM
## *The Way of Compassion*

# Tarthang Tulku, Rinpoche

*Question:* I'm a Buddhist and a therapist. I want to know how to be a good Buddhist therapist.

*Tarthang Tulku:* Therapy and Buddhism is a natural combination. In therapy the most important thing is compassion—not just giving explanations to the patient but giving yourself to him, trying to open your mind to him fully. Compassion is also the major focus of Buddhist practice, so Buddhism and therapy must always go together, again, not only to explain to the person so that he understands his problem but also to provide more self-givingness, more loving-kindness toward that person.

*Question:* How do I go about letting go of the ego and self, melting down and dissolving it?

*Answer:* It may not be necessary to melt the ego down if you understand it fully, if you understand that the ego is a part of the working process and that it is, in a way, necessary to enlightenment or to whatever goals you may have. It is true that our limited state of consciousness may be spoken of as egoistic. Nevertheless ego is necessary in order for us to attain any results or human goals. Therefore, although in religious or

philosophical terms what we call the ego is someth...
denied or done away with, or something to be transce...
nevertheless the first-level ego—not the selfish ego, but the
self-maintaining awareness—is necessary and should be kept
alive, even though Buddhism emphasizes that ego is the root
and cause of samsara. In a way, the ego is our projection. You
learn about yourself from it. It's like your own growth. So the
more you watch the ego, the more you learn. Therefore, in the
beginning, ego should not be wiped out.

*Question:* Could you tell me in your words the feeling you get
from nirvana?

*Answer:* Nirvana is very complicated, because Buddhism is
very complicated and very sophisticated; it is not easy to make
it into something simple. But the idea of nirvana is the idea of
full enlightenment, which means freedom from all bondages or
problems, whether on the physical, mental, or emotional level.
   Interpretation of the term nirvana is difficult because we
always project our viewpoint. Whatever we say, it is subjective, it is the way we feel it. And this is usually the way we
philosophize. If we do not forget this fact about the limitations
of interpretation, we may say that nirvana is complete freedom from samsara, which means, again, freedom from all
bondage.

*Question:* What assumption does the Buddhist therapist have
to make about himself and about his patient?

*Answer:* The Buddhist therapist must understand the human
mind intellectually, plus he must understand *himself,* how his
own mind works. Whatever form of human behavior he is
faced with, he has the possibility of a deeper understanding,
which can come from his religious practices. He must understand how the total human mind works, how it reacts, what
the consequences are, the emotional levels, the positive and

nds how the mind works experien-
ording to the Scriptures alone. This
of inward study and inner depth.

the relationship in Buddhism between
nt?

et there are four major schools, the earliest is
ca        ma. Like all the schools, the Nyingma has
develo    a system of inner practice, which is passed on
through oral instruction. Also there are a great many written
texts, a vast body of literature. These texts categorize all
human beings under nine classifications. Each person at any
given moment manifests a specific level of awareness. The
master or teacher or therapist is a person who can understand
each level of human consciousness both through his own
experience as well as through having received oral instruction.
Such an extraordinary person cannot mistreat another human
being; there are no gaps between him and another person. He
can put himself totally in the place of the patient. In other
words, he is not treating somebody else; in a way, he is treating
himself. There is no discrimination.

*Question:* What is karma?

*Answer:* Karma is the idea of cause and effect. Karma is, in a
way, all action, any human action and any kind of action—
even if I move my hand, that also is part of karma. Karma is
not necessarily the idea that in past lifetimes I have done some
good things which make me happy in this life, or that I caused
suffering and therefore I have bad experiences now. This is the
common view of karma, but it's not complete. Basically karma
means the law of inner causality. The Buddha explains that
everything is basically cause and effect. So the consequences of
our whole world, your world, my world, and all beings, are all
explained by karma.

*Question:* I know practically nothing about Tibetan Buddhism. What is so unique about your brand of Tibetan Buddhism and what does it have to offer me or other people here in California?

*Answer:* Buddhism may be summarized into three schools basic to Asian countries. First, there was Hinayana, which now flourishes in Ceylon and Southeast Asia. Then in northern India, China, Mongolia, and Japan, Mahayana Buddhism took root; later on, there began the esoteric practice, which is called Vajrayana. These three yanas—these three teachings—have all been preserved in Tibetan Buddhism.

In my opinion, which may not necessarily be true, there are several things Tibetan Buddhism can contribute that are unique. One of the most important is the range of its psychology. Western psychology, although it is very practical in certain aspects, is not fully comprehensive. It has not yet discovered the full potential of the human mind. In this area, Buddhism has much to contribute, and there is already a very healthy interest in Tibetan Buddhism on the part of some Western psychologists and mental-health professionals.

In addition, although Western psychology has many techniques and interesting theories, it offers nothing that can directly transmute human problems through a sort of recycling of psychic energy. Everyone either fights his problem or denies it or tries to avoid it. There is no way to use the energy generated by human emotional problems or neuroses. In those areas, particularly, I think Vajrayana, the esoteric part of the Buddha's teachings, can help tremendously. The key to most of the problems of human life on earth lies in understanding the human mind. We always feel our problems can be solved in an external way, but almost all our problems are in reality manifestations of our human mind. So therefore, in dealing with these situations, it is necessary to understand directly the entire reach of the mind. In this, Vajrayana, or esoteric Buddhism, reflects the understanding of the early traditions.

*Question:* How would you define health and disease and the phenomenon of healing?

*Answer:* There are many different techniques in healing. One person may have developed the way of visualization; another, chanting of mantras; or still another, the way of meditation. There are various ways through use of these various devotional channels. We tend to believe a healer is someone special, who is indispensable. He can heal me and solve my problems. But I think that the essential healing can be done by oneself. For example, if you have a physical or mental problem, breathe deeply and relax completely. This is just the elementary level, but as beginners we need to feel the sensations that accompany real relaxation. Once you are completely relaxed, both physically and mentally, there is a feeling of calmness; and that calm relaxation increases some sort of inner energy, which you yourself can develop and continue to increase. This healing energy can be useful for many purposes in our everyday conflicting emotions and human problems. Once you get this feeling, you eventually reach the state where you no longer have a self-identity; the tenseness of the ego is gone, you don't feel you possess a self, and you become a part of the relaxation. The relaxation feeds you, it transforms you; and you experience the state of what the religious sometimes call "samadhi," or "bliss." This healing we can generate from our mind and physical body. And this is different from someone who has particular healing techniques.

If you try to relax for a short time every day as much as you can, then a sort of sensation or feeling will begin to arise and gradually turn into something very wonderful, like a healer. When thoughts of resentment rise, or anything with which you are not comfortable, you yourself can heal them. More and more you can eliminate your internal enemies; for example, we call anger an enemy, or frustration an enemy, but all our negativities can become part of the relaxation. In other words, real relaxation releases energy that can be used to heal ourselves.

*Question:* How does that relate to what you spoke of before—the difference between *solving* a problem, which is the aim of Western psychotherapy, and using the energy to transform the problem, which is the aim of Vajrayana?

*Answer:* We are all beginners who are trying to find inner truth. We must begin slowly and gradually, step by step, to transcend all the negativities. It is not something we can do in one immediate step. However, we can definitely learn something when we have problems or difficulties. At that particular moment, just relax. Energy itself becomes transformed.

*Question:* What is the cause of the rising of indignation at an external object and what are the factors that would lead to not expressing that indignation?

*Answer:* My perceptions are automatically registered through my senses and through my mental conditioning. My subjective activity reacts, responds, and communicates with objects, so there is always an interrelationship in which the reaction is instant, automatic. Ordinarily, people cannot easily cope with this or cannot immediately transcend or change it. However, there is a way you can deal with it directly the moment it comes. If, in the present moment of experience, you can go directly toward the meditative state, then there are no longer any subject-object relationships you need to find out about, for these are all results of intellectual speculation. The important thing here is that you don't need to know very much about causes, whether internal or external. These are simply explanations offered by the thinking mind. But very practically, when the situation arises, just sit there and be the way you are, and completely cope with that experience of how you are in the moment. That is a task requiring skill. All samsaric problems, no matter what they are, are very useful; were there no problems there could be neither nirvana nor bodhisattvas. So solving samsaric or human mental problems is a learning process that brings self knowledge. Whether internal or external, this direct participation in my own problems is the best source of knowledge.

*Question:* Can a man be enlightened without a teacher, and, if he can, must he go out and teach others?

*Answer:* Yes, he can without a teacher—yes, it's possible. Buddhism has many traditions, so someone may also say, no, you can't, you must have a teacher. But in the overall view, I think there are definitely exceptions, and historically, there have been such people. There is no Buddha, there is no teacher. The best sort of teacher is self-awareness, inner intelligence. So if the person is very intelligent he may not necessarily have to go through the traditional way. Practice is all.

*Question:* If a man *is* enlightened and does it on his own, is it necessary for him to teach others?

*Answer:* It has been many, many generations since Lord Buddha—twenty-five hundred years—and yet the human condition is still with us. Even though the Buddha *is* a good person, he *is* intelligent, he *is* really a dynamic teacher, still he cannot completely solve all human conditions and problems. Therefore, there is always a need for continuation. Also, there are many other sentient beings. The Buddhist cosmos is much bigger and broader than we can see or believe.

*Question:* Western culture is becoming more interested in Eastern culture, and Eastern culture is becoming more Western. Do you think there will be a mutual evolution?

*Answer:* I think the majority of Easterners are becoming more interested in the materialistic level, in external forms. I do not wish to seem fault-finding, but among Easterners there doesn't seem to be as much internal development in the present era. Rather, their attention is focused on fulfilling external human desires. Human desires generate all objects and all existence, so this is seen as beautiful, and there is attraction. Therefore, many Easterners, particularly the younger generations, look at developments in the West and think they are seeing an absolute sort of solution.

On the other hand, Westerners have become interested in Eastern thought. The West has gone through many different stages and many different levels. Westerners have had a sort of comprehensive experience and have been tremendously involved on the samsaric level, inwardly and outwardly. So they have accumulated a great deal of knowledge for solving human problems on the materialistic level. They have reached something but now realize it is not an absolute answer. That is the reason they have become more interested in inner searching. They are seriously looking for something that has more significance, and I think this searching will have a world-wide influence if the West can develop its own resources toward inner research.

*Question:* What do you think is the significance of something so ancient being brought here now?

*Answer:* You may have heard about the great saint Padmasambhava. He predicted that in this century Westerners would be searching more within themselves. And I think this really seems the right time, particularly in America, and especially here in California, where we have a reputation for always searching for something. There is something genuinely interesting going on now, which means people here have a tremendously broad knowledge and are becoming more interested in every aspect of knowledge, wherever they can get it.

It is not because of Buddhist teachings alone, or only Indian or other Eastern philosophies. But I think this searching will reach the point where people discover that some of the Eastern thought and Western research are the same. Perhaps we will call the similarities Eastern, but it's not necessarily Eastern knowledge only. Westerners also have their own tradition, and they have learned quite a lot. It seems that both are reaching the same point at the same time.

*Question:* What does Buddhism mean by the idea that there is no ego? Sometimes I feel I seek enlightenment only to see my own ego in operation, rather than because I feel it is possible for me to become enlightened.

*Answer:* There are several levels of ego. In respect to the first level of ego, we believe there is something concrete, something solid which is within each person. However, if we directly examine this individualistic part of man, or ego-centeredness, we find there is not really anything substantial there. But that doesn't necessarily mean we cannot become enlightened and also function well. Actually, the more one gains the enlightening experience, the better one is able to function. But one must have knowledge. Knowledge can become a substitute for one's own self-grasping ego. So knowledge itself—one's self knowledge—becomes part of the ego or, one may say, one's own awareness. This knowledge takes care of everything and becomes enlightenment. So he who is enlightened is also self-sustained or self-reliant.

*Question:* How did you come to know of your reincarnations?

*Answer:* Philosophically, according to Buddhism, my mind, or this consciousness at its root, does not seem to come from the hundred or so chemical elements, or from whatever scientists say existence is. Therefore, there must be something beyond that, some background. Also, the other premise is that death is not just a physical body dying but is constantly going on—evolution is constantly starting—every single moment. So what does the mind contain? The past? My past is already gone, but the present is still functioning. And who is functioning? If the past is completely past, and the past is not present, then what is functioning? Who is the thread, the continuation —who is supposedly *that?* So therefore, it is believed that underlying consciousness there is definitely continuation.

*Question:* What means are available to us in the West to learn about our past lives?

*Answer:* Well, past lives are reflected in the present. If you take the past as completely separate, it becomes fragmented, cut off from possible knowledge. But at the same time, on another level, the illusions of our habit patterns are continually functioning. If you can transcend the present, then past and present become one thing.

*Question:* Is it the karma that is reborn or is it the consciousness?

*Answer:* Karma involves the process of developing—it is the product or result. It is stimulated, cultivated. But the consciousness, the cause, is reborn. The continuation is the consciousness. Consciousness has many flavors, sometimes at an unknown level, and it covers a lot of territory. Some Buddhist philosophers explain the entire universe as a projection of consciousness. Within ourselves, we perhaps make dialogues—this is subject, this is object. For example, at nighttime I have problems, something I don't like—I see it, I grasp it, I deny it, I discriminate, or whatever. I have separate things happening within the dream. In the morning I wake up. The subject, I, *was* there, but now I am here. But this is all *one* dream. There is no separate object and subject. So the same situation: once you get beyond the human consciousness level, both object and subject become unified. There is no separateness left. This is a theory. But there are practical aspects; you have to develop gradually into that stage—you can't just quickly jump there.

*Question:* How do you treat people diagnosed as schizophrenics?

*Answer:* The best way to treat people is not to make them suspicious of you. Do not create extra problems. The more you label their problem, the more it is increased. So the best way is to treat them as normal. In other words, a good psychologist will not act as if there were something wrong or different about the patient.

*Question:* I was thinking about when you put people in special environments.

*Answer:* I see. Well, in Tibet there is a wonderful quality of environment. There is enough space. Enough so that no individual is crowded, so there is no tension, no pressure. The farmer in America, for example, doesn't have such mental illness. There may be sickness, but it is very rare because the atmosphere stimulates one's energies and keeps one free from blockages. I think perhaps the schizophrenic—although there are many different types, of course—may not be so terribly bad, because he has his own way of observing and his own way of being. If he can simply function properly, he can be useful. Sometimes we can make a mistake, so that by treating such a person in one way we make it worse instead of helping.

*Question:* Some people speak of the difficulty, almost the impossibility, of transmitting meaning to another person. Now, a little earlier tonight I heard you mention the word *compassion.* Could you comment on the system or the systemization of compassion?

*Answer:* Buddha activity means compassion. And what is its purpose? Let us say you achieve enlightenment; does that mean there is nothing left for you to do? We say that until all sentient beings become enlightened you have a purpose. In fact, the purpose of my becoming enlightened is for the sake of all sentient beings, not for the sake of myself.

For example, in Buddhism one's parents are very important and Buddhism asks us to consider intently how much struggling most of our parents have gone through in order to give us the best they could offer and in order to see us through childhood. But we see that on the whole we never remember that, we only take selfishly without giving back anything. Now, taking that further, Buddhism teaches that you are the parent of all sentient beings countless numbers of times, and they in turn have been your parents as well; everything is extraordinarily interrelated.

As one realizes this, each relationship becomes based on feelings of love—not calculated love, but a natural friendliness to all beings, a natural openness based on a natural understanding of interrelationship. Gradually, the whole idea of *self*-motivation disappears, and one sees that when you have no self-motivation or self-interest, then all of your own problems get solved. There no longer exists any individual problem.

Of course, that is a far aim. But in terms of Buddhist psychology and therapy, we can see it this way. Everywhere and with everyone problems exist all of the time. There are all kinds of problems, a tremendous amount of suffering in the world. But the basic human problem is the same everywhere. The more I learn of other problems, the more my own problem automatically dissolves. So it is important to observe other people's problems, not just my own. And, if I can respond compassionately to other people's suffering, communication becomes a healing link that operates in both directions. At the same time, the more we understand other people, the more instantaneous and automatic is the compassionate response.

All of this is the beginning of real openness. The more open you become, the fewer problems you have. You are dedicated to all sentient beings, which is part of the idea of the bodhisattva. Knowledge of the other person increases self knowledge; self knowledge increases compassion; compassion increases knowledge of the other person. It is a very tight circle which can only be entered through giving up excessive preoccupation with one's own problems.

*Question:* Do you consider meditation as the foundation for the development of awareness?

*Answer:* Yes, definitely, meditation is just that. There may be times in the very deep stages of meditation, I think, when a person may experience something like darkness, or blackness, or a sort of numb state; but one eventually goes through this state to a greatly heightened awareness.

These are interesting things. When we have a meditation experience, we always feel so important: "I have a meditation experience!" After all, we have gone through so much trouble getting the experience.

But eventually the experience becomes part of the fixation, part of the shell, part of the problem—we are still living in our own world. If we can break that shell, then thoughts, concepts, blockages, and so on, automatically dissolve. In other words, the best meditation is *non*experience. But that is at a tremendously higher level of consciousness; it's not at our level. On this level we have to get some experience, but eventually we have to get beyond the experiential center. Only then will we experience a truly clear awareness.

*Question:* Can you say something about the practice of Vajrayana Buddhism?

*Answer:* The practice of Vajrayana Buddhism is a very big subject. But if you do meditation, develop your concentration as much as you can, and gradually move it within every thought, thought itself is practice. You know, our immediate question is, "What do I do with my thoughts?" But you can meditate within thought. Don't beat the thought itself, don't try to ignore it. Just sit inside the thought. Expand it, and the thought itself becomes meditation. This is more or less the basic foundation of the Vajrayana idea. Any thought, any feeling, any discrimination you may have, expand it. From this, the thought has its own particular field or space, and you can expand it completely. There are no longer any demanding levels.

*Question:* Is Vipassana° a Vajrayana practice?

*Answer:* Vipassana is basically a Theravada practice. You can use that also. Concentration comes first. You concentrate on your breath, or inhaling, or hearing; just breathing, very calm. These are among the various beginning techniques, but eventually you need to develop all the feelings or thoughts.

*Question:* My friend has what our society would consider a beautiful life: a big house, money in the bank, and a well-paying job. The whole economy is in such trouble one feels a tendency to go after and hold on to such things. At the same time there is an urge to pursue the spiritual life and give up this kind of life, which during these times would seem a crazy thing to do. What about this?

*Answer:* It doesn't matter what you have. Whether you're wealthy or whether you're poor, you need to appreciate it. Enjoy it. Be completely satisfied. Whatever you have, whether it be a small portion or a big portion, you must learn to appreciate it. The human mind is very interesting. We think, "This is my whole hindrance. If I give this up, then I will have

° The practice of mindfulness, or being aware of oneself in all conditions of living.

no more problems." But when I reach that place, internally all the same activities are still going on. So therefore just use whatever you have without grasping or trying to attract attention. Enjoy whatever things you have and transform them into meditation. It's possible to expand emotional-physical sensations to the point where you go beyond them. So whatever you have, enjoy it to the fullest, really to the fullest. Do not use it selfishly and don't make guilt feelings, but just live within the meditation.

*Question:* It seems to me that the way one begins on the Buddhist path is by analyzing one's mind. What texts can guide Westerners along this path of self-analysis?

*Answer:* A vast amount of the ancient teachings, a vast amount of knowledge, has been translated into Tibetan. The original Tripitaka,° for instance, contain more than five hundred volumes and many, many commentaries. But in the West, the available materials are very elementary, just a beginning. Gradually we hope to translate the really useful texts. There are some very convincing books, in a psychological way, that seem to clear up and completely solve all one's problems. Gradually we want to translate them, but it takes time and energy. At present there are only a few, such as Herbert Guenther's work. Lama Govinda's work is also interesting, and some other people have written introductions to Tibetan Buddhism. You can read some of these things and get an idea and a feeling of some of the practices. Also there is Evans-Wentz's work, but these various writings on Tibetan Buddhism have not been translated in an orderly fashion. Some of them seem to be random parts and sections, so they should not be there—but it is already done. Certain texts should be translated first, in an orderly fashion, but this has not yet been done. We are getting more facilities and more people are

° The Three Baskets (Collections) of the Pali Canon, the earliest Buddhist Scriptures.

learning the Tibetan language, so eventually we ourselves can do the translating. But at present I can't recommend very many beginning books. If you are religiously inclined, then perhaps *The Jewel Ornament of Liberation*° would be helpful. And from the psychologist's viewpoint, perhaps Lama Govinda's books. Also, Dr. Guenther has recently translated *Mind in Buddhist Psychology,*† and that too is very elementary.

*Question:* What is the difference between a meditating mind and a brooding mind?

*Answer:* Meditating is complete openness. The other is a blockage. The meditator has no specific blockage but just complete openness—no longer belonging to, or suppressing, or ignoring, or escaping. It's not hypnosis or the hypnotic state, and it's not just struggling, struggling until finally you just give up—until "there's no thought"—it's not that way. It is just completely clear and calm, and absolutely fresh. The mind is very fresh.

*Question:* What are mantras? Is mantra a form of self-hypnotism?

*Answer:* No. There are four or five things for which we cannot give logical explanations, such as the mantra, beauty, art, medicine, and samadhi. There aren't any logical answers as to why or how it works, but the mantra is some sort of energy. There is, broadly speaking, some higher energy that opens the mind instead of closing it down as with self-hypnosis. With most words we use there is always some kind of labeling. Each word draws forth some image or has some meaning within our consciousness. But the mantra has no such distractions. One simply listens to the mantra, concentrates on it, and becomes part of it; then there is nothing other than the mantra. It is a

° sGam. po. pa., Shambhala, Berkeley, California, 1971.
† Dharma Publishing, Emeryville, California, 1975.

transforming process, like music. The music, the instruments, and the person—each individually may not be beautiful, but the combination creates a wonderful feeling of joy or of something happening internally. This experience also comes through chanting the mantra.

*Question:* What is your main goal in life?

*Answer:* My main goal, my really deepest main goal, is to help, to be of service to someone. I may not always be successful in my service to others, or I may not know the best way; but if I successfully reach that goal, then I will be of service to everyone.

*Question:* Could you share with us a little information about the other lamas from Tibet and what's happening? Where are they?

*Answer:* There are very many lamas who fled to India as refugees. There may be ten thousand students there but very few masters. Some of these lamas are very learned and very intellectual, also very physically or spiritually achieved, and highly respected. They have problems, too—the problems of communication, the language problem, the aging problem, the distance problem; and also, India itself is not that interested. Even though there is much knowledge there, it is not of much use. Also, some of the young Tibetan students are more involved in earning a livelihood and have become more interested in the samsaric way than in their own tradition. But there are many lamas who live in the Himalayas, in Nepal, in Bhutan and Sikkim and throughout India who wish to come to the West. We hope to have a Country Center in the future where they can have a quiet place to stay and to teach. [Since this talk was given, land has been purchased in northern California, and construction is under way.] This is one of my projects. There are conditions and obstacles to be overcome, but I am trying to get a few teachers here who can share some of their knowledge.

*Question:* Did you know Thomas Merton and could you tell us some of the things about Tibet that inspired him the most?

*Answer:* He said that if he had a chance he would like to study the Nyingma for the rest of his life.

*Question:* Are there any common symbols that could have meaning in all religions so that we don't divide ourselves up into games or a fight for our identities?

*Answer:* That depends very much on each individual, because each person relates to different symbols according to his own background or culture; some symbols are familiar but other ones are not. It is difficult to have a universal symbol. Even if there were a universal symbol, people would make their own interpretations. The use of a symbol—whatever you learn, the concepts, all the words, the language, the intellectuality, everything—only reaches up to a certain point. The point of the symbol, the reality behind it, gets forgotten. This is true in almost all religions or any higher philosophy; the speculation sort of stops and does not go beyond the symbol. But it is only there—beyond the symbol—that all religions agree and perhaps have the same goal.

*Question:* You say that having a good healthy ego is an important thing in embarking on an esoteric path; and yet you also say that self-motivation interferes with or gets in the way of esoteric efforts. What is the distinction between ego and self-motivation?

*Answer:* First, if I refer to the self, I do not necessarily refer to it in a negative sense. That self is used in a positive sense. Ego is still more inclined toward samsaric activity, denoting grasping or identifying. In a way they are related. But if you are a practitioner—if you practice meditation—there is still the fact that you are hungry, you have to take care of yourself, you have to work and help other people; these all require some sort of motivation. The more you clear the mind, the more motivation increases; and that motivation becomes more selfless and healthy. The ego way is more selfish—just me—the fearful or grasping way of identifying.

*Question:* During the time you have been working here with Americans, have you noticed any particular problems or any particular strengths that we have in this kind of work as opposed to Easterners?

*Answer:* Well, I really believe that in certain ways Westerners are better than the Easterners. I'm not trying to flatter you, but I think that Westerners have an openness and acceptance on a general level, particularly in California. It may not be deep, we don't know; but there is an acceptance here in America which doesn't exist in some Eastern countries. I think this is very special and that America has great potential. This is a positive statement. Then the other side is that the interest changes so quickly. In the East interest becomes stronger and it is not easy to change it. But here there are so many variations, so many changes.

*Question:* There is so much available here in California. What would you say would help one to recognize a real teacher?

*Answer:* There is only one way I can answer, and that is if the person is *really* compassionate. It doesn't even matter if he has right knowledge or not, as long as he is compassionate.

*Question:* Could you discuss briefly the use of the statues of the Buddha or bodhisattvas or lohans in the Buddhist tradition? Are they themselves a help toward transformation?

*Answer:* There are many myths and stories about how in some of the temples the statues actually come alive and talk to the students. There are many other interesting things in history too. In a sense, images may help. But Buddhism does not believe in those things. Yet at the same time there are many forms and figures of art objects, many deities, wrathful and peaceful and bodhisattva styles—particularly in the Vajrayana, or Tibetan, tradition. So if a particular person needs a certain deity or certain manifestation for his own meditation purposes, he uses it. That is the reason such objects are in the temple; but the statues themselves are not necessarily worshiped, as it may appear to people who do not understand their purpose. The statues are reminders of past teachers—like going back to the original source, the original idea—and are kept there symbolically. Some religions have no statues whatsoever, and some religions greatly emphasize them. I think both are very much the same, whether there is a figure or whether there is no figure. Some people are very interested on the physical level, in which case they may like to have contact with objects. In Christianity the father figure is very important. In Buddhism there are different figures. But the human mind always needs an image to associate with or relate to. It makes us feel good. So each person's method may be different. Truth has many different stages before the Absolute, and art objects may help one to find the truth.

*Question:* When you speak this word *mind,* you don't point to your head, you point to your solar plexus. Could you talk a little about this?

*Answer:* I think that the mind is not necessarily in one particular place physically. It is very peculiar. The mind, as soon as you talk or ask questions, becomes dispersed; it's no longer there. We are within there, or "who we are" is mind, or we are in the mind, or we are the mind. In the physical sense, we may have what we call chakras. There are different levels of chakras and different emotional centers, or mind centers. They can be, as you pointed out, the solar plexus, the head, or all these centers.

*Question:* Does Tibetan Buddhism attach special meanings to dreams, or do you think of them as shadows of samsara?

*Answer:* Yes. One of the six parts of Naropa's Doctrine has a section on dream yoga practices. The dream is part of Buddhism, particularly the Vajrayana tradition. Each one of these six stages of consciousness is different and yet interrelated. The dream is one stage, and then there is another stage. It is very important to know what the dream is.

*Question:* Do they have meanings and interpretations?

*Answer:* Yes, there are many different interpretations, but the interpretations are used more in psychology. However, the theory is that everything—all life—is like a dream.

*Question:* In the esoteric form of Buddhism, is there anything like devotion, faith, or worship, and if so, what of?

*Answer:* Yes and no. If you want to say yes, then that means devotion to whom? Yourself. And if you say no, then Buddhism does not necessarily believe in some protectors external to yourself.

*Question:* Is there a distinction in Buddhism between compassion, love, and helpfulness?

*Answer:* Yes. First is love. In the most common sense, love is self-motivation too; but this love is related to the physical sense, to sensations and feelings. This love has to do with feelings toward another and my expressing those feelings; so there is interaction. This love is on the first level. The second stage is sympathy and empathy, more like compassion. But compassion, as such, is more complete—there is no longer any self. There is no longer any grasping for yourself. Compassion is broader than love. Love is more on the consciousness level; compassion is more on the wisdom level. Helpfulness is used in both cases in one's regular activities. Helpfulness means you are responsible, you have a willingness, you are opening yourself.

*Question:* Would you believe that perhaps the best service that Buddhism and other Eastern thought can offer to the West, particularly Western therapy, is to get them to drop the whole concept and practice of therapy and just have compassionate people available to help people? And, isn't therapy almost by definition a suspicion-creating and guilt-creating process?

*Answer:* I don't think it is necessary to drop Western thoughts completely; but I think that if Western therapy provided more of the flavor of compassion, therapy would be more effective. Then therapy may become more enlightened; you create more beauty, more strength, something more meaningful. I think that Western psychotherapy also has something useful—some good observations—particularly in dealing with this culture, because it is your own heritage and your own custom. There is a certain way you can talk and communicate better with the patient. But there are also certain negative aspects that perhaps could be eliminated.

*Question:* Do you believe you live the philosophy of Buddha or do you live your own philosophy?

*Answer:* Whatever I have learned is part of Buddha's teachings, so most of what I am saying are Buddha's ideas. But some are definitely my own interpretations.

*Question:* What advice would you give to someone who came to you saying, "I'm very depressed, life has no meaning for me;

I'm thinking of killing myself, why should I live, why should I go on?"

*Answer:* Well, I can teach you how not to think like that. I can teach you that tomorrow is different from today, and that in the past you have constantly gone up and down, up and down. Therefore, you should not be discouraged with your life. If you are depressed now, you can be learning something about yourself; you can increase your self knowledge. And so I might also give you some advice about self-observation. And perhaps I would try to find out exactly who you really are. Maybe I would ask you directly, "What is the problem, actually? Is it really very serious?" If so, perhaps we can talk more; but usually the problems are really not that serious. Most of us just *think* we have a problem.

*Question:* Does mental illness invariably come about through lack of self-union?

*Answer:* Yes.

*Question:* You were talking about ups and downs, and I'm wondering if you get depressions.

*Answer:* Yes, but I don't give up.

*Question:* What are your specific ambitions in the operations of the Nyingma Institute?

*Answer:* First I want to establish more Abhidharma, which is the Buddhist psychology. And I want to bring as much Buddhist psychology into the West as possible; and to bring teachers and to make available more training and translations, such as the small book we recently published, *Mind in Buddhist Psychology.* Along this line I can spread more knowledge about what Buddhist psychology says about mind, about consciousness. After that, perhaps I will emphasize Madhyamika, which is the meditative philosophy. Everyone has vague ideas about enlightenment, so I want to provide a better description of the state of enlightenment—how it can be reached—and philosophize upon the whole idea of enlightenment. What is Sunyata? What is the Absolute? In this second stage I want to put more emphasis on these questions. The third stage is the Prajnaparamita. That describes more about what "Buddha" really means—the significance of the Buddha's enlightenment. The second stage is partial. The third one, the Prajnaparamita, is total, as Buddha really saw it—what reality is. Everything is part of the Buddha activity, Buddha nature. So I wish to explain these things more in sort of linguistic terms. Then eventually there will be Vajrayana practices.

I am not seeking to convince the West of how great Buddhism is. My aim is to present certain basic ideas of Buddhist philosophy, while emphasizing the practices, and then to unify both the practice and the philosophy. I do not mean for Buddhism to eliminate the Western therapies or religions; rather, I wish to integrate Buddhist ideas into your own culture and traditions to give them more strength. For example, I know many priests and psychologists for whom Buddhism has increased their understanding and interest in their own culture. The more you know about Buddhism, the more you can go back to your own culture. It works better both ways.

*Question:* From time to time a person will come up with new answers to old problems, like Einstein with the theory of relativity. How do you understand the creative process in Buddhism?

*Answer:* Among the Westerners attracted to Buddhism, some of the most interesting people have thought a great deal about the theory of relativity. Physicists in particular are intrigued by the Madhyamika philosophy, which agrees with much of modern physics, although using a very different kind of language. I like to work most of all with physicists and mathematicians. Buddhist ideas can be united with scientific knowledge and I think can aid tremendously in completely reconstructing world-wide knowledge.

*Question:* Do you think there is any adaptation necessary in Tibetan Buddhism to make it more suitable for the American scene?

*Answer:* This is a delicate situation. From the viewpoint of the Tibetans of serious traditional lineages, how much should we change, or could we change or not change? It is a difficult question. On the one hand, it seems necessary sometimes to change traditional Buddhist moral precepts and ideas. On the other hand, if we change them, then perhaps we will only be able to see how consciousness works on the surface level. In the long range, we can't predict this. It is simply too soon to give an answer to this question.

*Question:* What do you think of Trungpa Rinpoche and his activities?

*Answer:* I think what he is doing is very attractive and of tremendous interest to many people, but I think he is not necessarily completely following Tibetan traditions. But whether his is the best way or even perhaps the only way, I can't tell you. At present it can't be predicted.

*Question:* Can you explain the process of creation? Is it within the mind, a function of the mind? Where does a new thought, a new idea, come from?

*Answer:* I think sometimes new thoughts come from the past, from something like an archetypal mind. Certainly one occasionally makes contact with an unconscious level of mind where something can appear for which there is no conditioning—there is no explanation for it on the rational level. You can interpret such things and give explanations, but in the last analysis the mind is merely an operation. Things just happen—these old thoughts as well as new ideas.

*Question:* Is there a dialogue between Buddhism and Christian theology going on, and if so, at what points do they touch?

*Answer:* They come together on certain aspects of compassion or love and on morality too—sometimes. They also meet on the certainty of the presence of God, so to speak. On that level, they are very close sometimes.

*Question:* What are your views about sex and sexual morality?

*Answer:* I think the best sexual morality is complete relaxation.

*Question:* Do you think that using psychedelics in a disciplined way can be effective?

*Answer:* It depends very much on the individual. If the person has a great deal of knowledge in its use and also has a certain background in meditation and yoga, then perhaps it may help sometimes, but for the average person generally, I don't think so. Buddhist or spiritual masters always emphasize that naturalness is more important than any kind of technique. So in that sense it is not necessary to use it; but it depends.

*Question:* Were there any great women spiritual masters in this tradition, and if not, why not?

*Answer:* Yes, there are quite a few. There are a number of historical women, such as Padmasambhava's consort, Yeshe Tsogyal, who concealed all the secret documented teachings to preserve them. They call this the Terma tradition—treasures hidden all over the world. There are a number of very important women teachers too, even women reincarnations.

*Question:* You spoke earlier of the importance of compassion in psychotherapy. Do you see any difference in the various kinds of psychotherapy in terms of which has more compassion?

*Answer:* I think the person who is the best therapist is one who has himself gone beyond therapy. He no longer thinks in terms of therapy. If the person is no longer a "therapist," then he is a good therapist. That means he has great compassion. Some schools of thought may have more emphasis on compassion than others, but even though there are different schools and different traditions, it rests finally with the individual—some are more developed and are more actively compassionate than others.

*Question:* Are there specific mental and physical exercises that we can use to activate our healing influence?

*Answer:* I go back to the same thing I said earlier, that the best exercise I have found, and the simplest, is relaxation—of the mind, the breath, and the body. This is simple, not dangerous, and very effective and efficient. It is always there, so that you can use it anytime.

*Question:* You mentioned going into thought in meditation. Could you please elaborate on that a little bit?

*Answer:* Well, you can just take the present moment, keep your awareness there, and just be. And that becomes "going into thought." There are several dimensions in thought itself. I think I can see the thought, but one is not necessarily the seer, one is not necessarily separate from the thought. One is a part of thought. So as much as you can be in the present state, then you become meditation.

*Question:* Do you think it is necessary for all adepts or beginners to practice the preliminary hundred thousand prostrations?

*Answer:* This is designed particularly for someone who wants to go along the traditional path, but as I said before, it is not necessary for everyone to go the traditional way. A person may have had enough background and have already developed a great deal of self knowledge. It depends again on each individual.

*Question:* How do you judge?

*Answer:* It depends on how aware the person is, how much comprehension he has, how much he has developed his own consciousness, how he relates with other people, and how he deals with his own communication.

*Question:* Could you say something about the Vajrayana practice of visualization, and does the power of imagination play an active role in that?

*Answer:* Imagination is not the visualization; there is quite a marked difference between them. At first, we are only dealing with images which appear in imagination, which create imagination. Then, after we go beyond imagination, there are three-dimensional visualizations, such as beautiful heavens, beautiful images, beautiful figures, or beautiful concepts, which you can create beyond the human imagination realm. But these visualizations are specifically given by teachers to particular students who are interested in this kind of practice. This practice is also designed for specific cases where a person may have problems that he cannot solve in any other way.

Generally, ordinary people do not visualize. Only those who are going through a more specific form of training are given visualization practice.

*Question:* Many American people want money more than anything else and so have little time to practice. What compassion could you feel for Americans who are this way?

*Answer:* Compassion is very useful. You can have compassion for any type of person, even if the person is unreasonable or unjust to you; if he is not really wise, you can have compassion for his ignorance. You don't have to become personally involved on the physical level. But even if you have demanding situations, and there are lots of pressures, and people insist you have to act a certain way or you must be successful or else you will be nothing socially—society has many pressures—still you can be compassionate. Even though you are confronted with a very strong, demanding situation, you don't need to be angry with the person, but you have compassion for his ignorance. He simply is not aware of knowing.

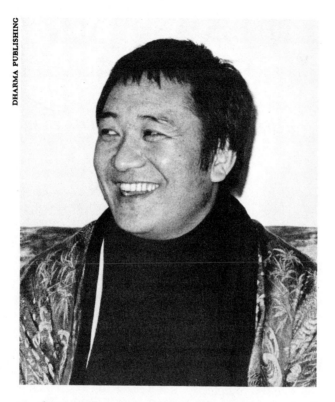

*Tarthang Tulku, Rinpoche,* is a reincarnate lama of the Tarthang monastery in Eastern Tibet. Since coming to America in 1969, he has established in Berkeley, California, the Tibetan Nyingmapa Meditation Center and the Nyingma Institute, centers for the study and practice of the ancient Tibetan tradition. His work in America has brought him into a live relationship both with numerous young people and with therapists, scientists, and artists throughout the country.

# PEAKS AND VALES

*The Soul / Spirit Distinction as Basis
for the Differences between
Psychotherapy and Spiritual Discipline*

## James Hillman

*The way through the world
Is more difficult to find than the way beyond it.
"Reply to Papini"*—WALLACE STEVENS

## I. IN SEARCH OF SOUL

Long ago and far away from California and its action, its concern, its engagement, there took place in Byzantium, in the city of Constantinople, in the year 869, a Council of the Principals of the Holy Catholic Church,[1] and because of their session then and another one of their sessions a hundred years prior (Nicaea, 787), we are all in this room tonight.

Because at that Council in Constantinople the soul lost its dominion. Our anthropology, our idea of human nature, devolved from a tripartite cosmos of spirit, soul, and body (or matter) to a dualism of spirit (or mind) and body (or matter). And this because at that other Council, the one in Nicaea in 787, images were deprived of their inherent authenticity.

We are in this room this evening because we are moderns in search of a soul, as Jung once put it. We are still in search of reconstituting that third place, that intermediate realm of psyche—which is also the realm of images and the power of imagination—from which we were exiled by theological, spiritual men more than a thousand years ago: long before Descartes and the dichotomies attributed to him, long before the Enlightenment and modern positivism and scientism. These ancient historical events are responsible for the malnourished root of our Western psychological culture and of the culture of each of our souls.

What the Constantinople Council did to soul only culminated a long process beginning with Paul, the Saint, of substituting and disguising, and forever after confusing, soul with spirit. Paul uses *psyche* only four times in his Epistles. *Psyche* appears in the entire New Testament only fifty-seven times compared with two hundred seventy-four occurrences of *pneuma*.[2] Quite a score! Of these fifty-seven occurrences of the word *psyche*, more than half are in the Gospels and Acts. The Epistles, the presentation of doctrine, the teachings of the school, could expose its theology and psychology without too much need for the word *soul*. For Paul four times was enough.

Much the same is true in regard to dreams and myths.[3] The word *to dream* does not appear in the New Testament; *dream* (*onar*) occurs only in three chapters of Matthew (1, 2, and 27). *Mythos* occurs only five times, pejoratively. Instead, there is stress on spirit phenomena: miracles, speaking in tongues, visions, revelations, ecstasy, prophecy, truth, faith.

Because our tradition has systematically turned against soul, we are each unaware of the distinctions between soul and spirit—therefore confusing psychotherapy with spiritual disciplines, obfuscating where they conflate and where they differ. This traditional denial of soul continues within the attitudes of each of us, whether Christian or not, for we are each unconsciously affected by our culture's tradition, the unconscious aspect of our collective life. Ever since Tertullian declared that the soul (anima) is naturally Christian, there has been a latent Christianity, an antisoul spirituality, in our Western soul. This has led eventually to a psychological disorientation, and we have had to turn to the Orient. We place, displace, or project into the Orient our Occidental disorientation. And my task in this lecture is to do what I can for soul. Part of this task, because it is ritualistically appropriate, is to point out C. G. Jung's part in prying loose the dead fingers of those dignitaries in old Turkey, both by restoring the soul as a primary experience and field of work and by showing us ways—particularly through images—of realizing that soul.

## II. PSYCHE AND IMAGE

The three hundred bishops assembled at Nicaea in 787 upheld the importance of images against the enemies of images, mainly the Imperial Byzantine army. Images were venerated and adored all through the antique world—statues, icons, paintings, and clay figures formed part of the local cults and were the focus of the conflict between Christianity and the old polytheistic religions. At the time of the Nicaean Council there had been another of those long battles between spirit and soul, between abstractions and images, between iconoclasts and idolaters, such as occur in the Bible and in the life of Mohammed, and such as occur in the Renaissance and in the Reformation when Cromwell's men broke the statues of Christ and Mary in the churches of England because they were the Devil's work and not Christian.

The hatred of the image, the fear of its power, and of the imagination, is very old and very deep in our culture.

Now, at Nicaea a subtle and devastating differentiation was made. Neither the imagists nor the iconoclasts got their way entirely. A distinction was drawn between the *adoration* of images and the free formulation of them on the one hand, and the *veneration* of images and the authorized control over them on the other.[4] Church Councils split hairs, but the roots of these hairs are in our heads, and the split goes deep indeed. At Nicaea a distinction was made between the image as such, its power, its full divine or archetypal reality, and what the image represents, points to, means. Thus, images became allegories.

When images become allegories the iconoclasts have won. The image itself has become subtly depotentiated. Yes, images are allowed, but only if they are officially approved images illustrative of theological doctrine.[5] One's spontaneous imagery is spurious, demonic, devilish, pagan, heathen. Yes, the image is allowed, but only to be venerated for what it represents: the abstract ideas, configurations, transcendences behind the image. Images became ways of perceiving doctrine, helps in focusing fantasy. They became representations, no longer presentations, no longer presences of the divine power.

The year 787 marks another victory in our tradition of spirit over soul. Jung's resuscitation of images was a return to soul and what he calls its spontaneous symbol formation, its life of fantasy (which, as he notes, is inherently tied with polytheism).[6] By turning to the image, Jung returned to the soul, reversing the historical process that in 787 had depotentiated images and in 869 had reduced soul to the rational intellectual spirit.

This is history, yet not only history. For each time you or I treat images as representations of something else—Penis, or Great Mother, or Power Drive, or Instinct, or whatever general, abstract concept we prefer—we have smashed the image in favor of the idea behind it. To give to imagination interpretative meanings is to think allegorically and to depotentiate the power of the imagination.

Here I want to remind you of Jung's position, from which I have developed mine. Jung's psychology is based on soul. It is a tripartite psychology. It is based neither on matter and the brain nor on the mind, intellect, spirit, mathematics, logic, metaphysics. He uses neither the methods of natural science and the psychology of perception nor the methods of metaphysical science and the logic of mentation. He says his base is in a third place between: *esse in anima,* "being in soul." [7] And he found this position by turning directly to the images in his insane patients and in himself during his breakdown years.

The soul and its images, having been alienated so long from

our conscious culture, could be recognized only by the alienist. (Or by the artist, for whom imagination and madness have always been kissin' cousins in our culture's anthropology.) So, Jung said, if you are in search of soul, go first to your fantasy images, for that is how the psyche presents itself directly.[8] All consciousness depends upon fantasy images. All we know about the world, about the mind, the body, about anything whatsoever, *including the spirit* and the nature of the divine, comes through images and is organized by fantasies into one pattern or another. This holds true also for such spiritual states as pure light, or the void, or absence, or merging bliss, each of which is captured or structured in soul according to one or another archetypal fantasy pattern.[9] Because these patterns are archetypal, we are always in one or another archetypal configuration, one or another fantasy, including the fantasy of soul and the fantasy of spirit. The "collective unconscious," which embraces the archetypes, means our unconsciousness of the collective fantasy that is dominating our viewpoints, ideas, behaviors, by means of the archetypes.

Let me continue for just a moment with Jung—though we are almost through the abstract, thinky part of this lecture—who says, "Every psychic process is an image and an imagining." [10] The only knowledge we have that is immediate and direct is knowledge of these psychic images. And further, when Jung uses the word *image*, he does not mean the reflection of an object or a perception; that is, he does not mean a memory or after-image. Instead he says his term is derived "from poetic usage, namely, a figure of fancy or fantasy image." [11]

This last should set sail to your minds: for Jung here suggests the poetic basis of consciousness, a consciousness based on primary givens which are poetic, or mythic, fantasy images. These do not come from "reality." In fact, says Jung, "The psyche creates reality every day. The only expression I can use for this activity is fantasy." [12]

I have spelled all this out because I want you to know what I am doing. I am showing how soul looks at spirit, how peaks look from the vale, from within the fantasy world that is the shifting structure of our consciousness and its formulations, which are always shaped by archetypal images. We are always in one or another root-metaphor, archetypal fantasy, mythic perspective. From the soul's point of view we can never get out of the vale of our psychic reality.

## III. SOUL AND SPIRIT

I have called this talk "Peaks and Vales," and I have been aiming to draw apart these images in order to contrast them as vividly as I can. Part of separating and drawing apart is the emotion of hatred. So I shall be speaking with hatred and urging strife, or *eris*, or *polemos*, which Heraclitus, the first ancestor of psychology, has said is the father of all.

The contemporary meaning of "peak" was developed by Abraham Maslow, who in turn was resonating an archetypal image, for peaks have belonged to the spirit ever since Mount Sinai and Mount Olympus, Mount Patmos and the Mount of Olives, and Mount Moriah of the first patriarchal Abraham. And you will easily name a dozen other mountains of the spirit. It does not require much explication to realize that the peak experience is a way of describing pneumatic experience, and that the clamber up the peaks is in search of spirit or is the drive of the spirit in search of itself. The language Maslow uses about the peak experience—"self-validating, self-justifying and carries its own intrinsic value with it," the God-likeness and God-nearness, the absolutism and intensity—is a traditional way of describing spiritual experiences. Maslow deserves our gratitude for having reintroduced *pneuma* into psychology, even if his move has been compounded by the old confusion of pneuma with psyche. But what about the *psyche* of psychology?

Vales do indeed need more exposition, just as everything to do with soul needs to be carefully imagined as accurately as we can. *Vale* comes from the Romantics: Keats uses the term in a letter, and I have taken this passage from Keats as a psychological motto: "Call the world, if you please, the vale of soul-making. Then you will find out the use of the world."

Vale in the usual religious language of our culture is a depressed emotional place—the vale of tears; Jesus walked this lonesome valley, the valley of the shadow of death. The very first definition of *valley* in the Oxford English Dictionary is a "long depression or hollow." The meanings of *vale* and *valley* include entire subcategories referring to such sad things as the decline of years and old age, the world regarded as a place of troubles, sorrow, and weeping, and the world regarded as the scene of the mortal, the earthly, the lowly.

There is also a feminine association with vales (unlike peaks). We find this in the Tao Te Ching, 6; in Freudian morphological metaphors, where the wooded river valley teeming with animal life is an equivalent for the vagina, and also we find a feminine connotation of the valley in mythology. For valleys are the places of the nymphs. One of the etymological explanations of the word *nymph* takes these figures to be personifications of the wisps and clouds of mist clinging to valleys, mountainsides, and water sources.[13] Nymphs veil our vision, keep us shortsighted, myopic, caught —no long-range distancing, no projections or prophecies as from the peak.

This peak/vale pairing is also used by the fourteenth Dalai Lama of Tibet. In a letter (to Peter Goullart) he writes:

> The relation of height to spirituality is not merely metaphorical. It is physical reality. The most spiritual people on this planet live in the highest places. So do the most spiritual flowers. . . . I call the high and light aspects of my being *spirit* and the dark and heavy aspect *soul.*
>
> Soul is at home in the deep, shaded valleys. Heavy torpid flowers saturated with black grow there. The rivers flow like warm syrup. They empty into huge oceans of soul.

Spirit is a land of high, white peaks and glittering jewel-like lakes and flowers. Life is sparse and sounds travel great distances.

There is soul music, soul food, soul dancing, and soul love. . . .

When the soul triumphed, the herdsmen came to the lamaseries, for soul is communal and loves humming in unison. But the creative soul craves spirit. Out of the jungles of the lamasery, the most beautiful monks one day bid farewell to their comrades and go to make their solitary journey toward the peaks, there to mate with the cosmos. . . .

No spirit broods over lofty desolation; for desolation is of the depths, as is brooding. At these heights, spirit leaves soul far behind. . . .

People need to climb the mountain not simply because it is there but because the soulful divinity needs to be mated with the spirit. . . . [abbreviated]

May I point out one or two little curiosities in this letter. They may help us to see further the contrast between soul and spirit. First, did you notice how important it is to be *literal* and not "merely metaphorical" when one takes the spiritual viewpoint? Also, this viewpoint requires the *physical sensation* of height, of "highs." Then, did you see that it is the most *beautiful* monks who leave their brothers, and that their mating is with the cosmos, a mating that is compared with snow? (Once in our witch-hunting Western tradition, a time obsessively concerned with protecting soul from wrong spirits —and vice versa—the devil was identified by his icy penis and cold sperm.) And finally, have you noticed the two sorts of *anima symbolism*: the dark, heavy, torpid flowers by the rivers of warm syrup and the virginal petaled flowers of the glaciers?

I am trying to let the *images* of language draw our distinction. This is the soul's way of proceeding, for it is the way of dreams, reflections, fantasies, reveries, and paintings.

We can recognize what is spiritual by its style of imagery and language; so with soul. To give *definitions* of spirit and soul—the one abstract, unified, concentrated; the other concrete, multiple, immanent—puts the distinction and the problem into the language of spirit. We would already have left the valley; we would be making differences like a surveyor, laying out what belongs to whom according to logic and law rather than according to imagination.

Let us turn to another culture a little closer to home even if far away in time: the early desert saints in Egypt, whom we might call the founders of our Western ascetic tradition, our discipline of the spirit.

We must first recall that these men were Egyptians, and as Violet MacDermott has shown,[14] their spiritual moves need to be understood against their Egyptian religious background. As the inheritor of an enduring polytheistic religion, the desert saint attempted to "reverse the psychological effects of the ancient religion." His discipline aimed to separate the monk from his human community and also from nature, both of which were of vital importance to the polytheistic religion in which divine and human interpenetrated everywhere (that is, in the valley, not only at the peak or the desert). By living in a cave—the burial place of the old religion—the desert saint performed a mimesis of death: the rigors of his spiritual discipline, its peculiar postures, fasting, insomnia, darkness, etc. These rigors helped him withstand the assault of the demons, or ancestral influences of the dead, as well as his personal and cultural history.

> The world of the Gods was, in Egypt, also the world of the dead. Through dreams, the dead communicated with the living . . . therefore sleep represented a time when his soul was subject to his body and to those influences which derived from his old religion . . . his ideal was to sleep as little as possible.[15]

Again you will have noticed the turn away from sleep and dreams, away from nature and community, away from personal and ancestral history and polytheistic complexity. These factors from which the spiritual discipline works to be free give specific indications about the nature of the soul.

We find another contrast between soul and spirit, couched in different terms from the spiritual ones we have been examining, in E. M. Forster's little volume *Aspects of the Novel*, in which he lays out the basic components of the art of the novel. He makes a distinction between fantasy and prophecy. He says that both involve mythology, Gods. Then he calls up fantasy with these words:

> . . . let us now invoke all beings who inhabit the lower air, the shallow water, and the smaller hills, all Fauns and Dryads and slips of the memory, all verbal coincidences, Pans and puns, all that is medieval this side of the grave [by which I guess him to mean the coarse, common, and humorous, the daily, the grotesque and freakish, even bestial, but also festive].[16]

When Forster comes to prophecy we gain yet more images of spirit, for prophecy in the novel pertains

> to whatever transcends our abilities, even when it is human passion that transcends them, to the deities of India, Greece, Scandinavia, and Judea, to all that is medieval beyond the grave and to Lucifer son of the morning [by which last I take him to mean the "problem of good and evil"]. By their mythologies we shall distinguish these two sorts of novels.[17]

By their mythologies we shall also distinguish our therapies.

Forster goes on with the comparison, but we shall break off, taking only a few scattered observations. Spirit (or the prophetic style) is humble but humorless. "It may imply any of the faiths that have haunted humanity—Christianity, Buddhism, dualism, Satanism, or the mere raising of human love and hatred to such a power that their normal receptacles no longer contain them." [18] (You recall the lama mating with the cosmos, the desert saint alone.) Prophecy (or spirit) is mainly a tone of voice, an accent, such as we find in the novels of D. H. Lawrence and Dostoevsky. Fantasy (or soul, in my terms) is a wondrous quality in daily life. "The power of fantasy penetrates into every corner of the universe, but not into the forces that govern it—the stars that are the brain of heaven, the army of unalterable law, remain untouched—and novels of this type have an improvised air. . . ." [19] Here I think of the free associations of Freud as a *method* in psychology, or of Jung's mode of writing where no paragraph logically follows the one preceding, or of Lévi-Strauss's figure, the *"bricoleur,"* the handyman and his ragtag putting together of collages, and how different this psychological style is from that of intensely focused transcendental meditation, the turning away, the emptying out.

And finally for our purposes Forster says about fantasy novels, or soul-writing, "If one god must be invoked specially, let us call upon Hermes—messenger, thief, and conductor of souls. . . ." [20]

Forster points to something else about soul (by means of his notion of fantasy), and this something else is *history*. The soul involves us in history—our individual case history, the history of our therapy, our culture as history. (We have seen the Coptic ascetics attempting to overcome ancestral history through spiritual practices.) Here, I too am speaking soul language in going back all the time to historical examples, such as old E. M. Forster, little fussy man in his room in Cambridge, now dead, and dead Freud and Jung, back to old myths and their scholarship, to etymologies and the history in words, and down to specific geographical localities, the actual vales of the world. For this is the way the soul proceeds. This is psychological method, and psychological method remains within this valley world, through which history passes and leaves its traces, our "ancestors."

The peaks wipe out history. History is to be overcome. History is bunk, said Henry Ford, prophetic manufacturer of obsolescence, and the past is a bucket of ashes, said Carl Sandburg, prophetic singer. So the spirit workers and spirit seekers first of all must climb over the debris of history, or prophesy its end or its unreality, time as illusion, as well as the history of their individual and particular localities, their particular ethnic and religious roots (Jung's ill-favored earlier term "racial unconscious"). Thus, from the spirit point of view, it can make no difference if our teacher be a Zaddik from a Polish shtetl, an Indian from under a Mexican cactus, or a Japanese master in a garden of stones; these differences are but conditionings of history, personalistic hangups. The spirit is impersonal, rooted not in local soul, timeless.

I shall ride this horse of history until it drops, for I submit that history has become the Great Repressed. If in Freud's time sexuality was the Great Repressed and the creator of the internal ferment of the psychoneuroses, today the one thing we will not tolerate is history. No; we are each Promethean with a bag of possibilities, Pandoran hopes, open; unencumbered, the future before us, so various, so beautiful, so new—new and liberated men and women living forward into a science fiction. So history rumbles below, continuing to work in our psychic complexes.

Our complexes are history at work in the soul: father's socialism, his father's fundamentalism, and my reaction against them like Hefner to Methodism, Kinsey to Boy-Scoutism, Nixon to Quakerism. It is so much easier to transcend history by climbing the mountain and let come what may than it is to work on history within us, our reactions, habits, moralities, opinions, symptoms that prevent true psychic change. Change in the valley requires recognition of history, an archaeology of the soul, a digging in the ruins, a re-collecting. And—a planting in specific geographical and historical soil with its own smell and savor, in connection with the spirits of the dead, the *po*-soul sunk in the ground below.

125

From the viewpoint of soul and life in the vale, going up the mountain feels like a desertion. The lamas and saints "bid farewell to their comrades." As I'm here as an advocate of soul, I have to present its viewpoint. Its viewpoint appears in the long hollow depression of the valley, the inner and closed dejection that accompanies the exaltation of ascension. The soul feels left behind, and we see this soul reacting with anima resentments. Spiritual teachings warn the initiate so often about introspective broodings, about jealousy, spite, and pettiness, about attachments to sensations and memories. These cautions present an accurate phenomenology of how the soul feels when the spirit bids farewell.

If a person is concurrently in therapy and in a spiritual discipline—Vedanta, breathing exercises, transcendental meditation, etc.—the spiritual teacher may well regard the analysis as a waste of time with trivia and illusions. The analyst may regard the spiritual exercises as a leak in the psychic vessel, or an escape into either physicality (somatizing, a sort of sophisticated hysterical conversion) or into metaphysicality. These are conditions that grow in the same hedgerow, for both physicalize, substantiate, hypostasize, taking their concepts as things. They both lose the "as if," the metaphorical Hermes approach, forgetting that metaphysics too is a fantasy system, even if one that must unfortunately take itself as literally real.

Besides these mutual accusations of triviality, there is a more essential question that we in our analytical armchairs ask: *Who is making the trip?* Here it is not a discussion about the relative value of doctrines or goals; nor is it an analysis of the visions seen and experiences felt. The essential issue is not the analysis of content of spiritual experiences, for we have seen similar experiences in the county hospital, in dreams, in drug trips. Having visions is easy. The mind never stops oozing and spurting the sap and juice of fantasy, and then congealing this play into paranoid monuments of eternal truth. And then are not these seemingly mind-blowing events of light, of synchronicity, of spiritual sight in an LSD trip often trivial—seeing the universe revealed in a buttonhole stitch or linoleum pattern— at least as trivial as what takes place in a usual therapy session that picks apart the tangles of the daily domestic scene?

The question of what is trivial and what is meaningful depends on the archetype that gives meaning, and this, says Jung, is the self. Once the self is constellated, *meaning* comes with it. But as with any archetypal event, it has its undifferentiated foolish side. So one can be overwhelmed by displaced, inferior, paranoid meaningfulness, just as one can be overwhelmed by eros and one's soul (anima) put through the throes of desperate, ridiculous love. The disproportion between the trivial content of a synchronistic event on the one hand, and on the other, the giant sense of meaning that comes with it, shows what I mean. Like a person who has fallen into love, so a person who has fallen into meaning begins that process of self-validation and self-justification of trivia which belong to the experience of the archetype within any complex and form part of its defense. It therefore makes little difference, psychodynamically, whether we fall into the shadow and justify our disorders of morality, or the anima and our disorders of beauty, or the self and our disorders of meaning. Paranoia has been defined as a disorder of meaning—that is, it can be referred to the influence of an undifferentiated self archetype. Part of this disorder is the very systematization that would, by defensive means of the doctrine of synchronicity, give profound meaningful order to a trivial coincidence.

Here we return to Mr. Forster, who reminded us that the spirit's voice is humble and the soul's humorful.[21] Humility is awed and wowed by meaning; the soul takes the same events more as the puns and pranks of Pan.[22] Humility and humor are two ways of coming down to *humus,* to the human condition. Humility would have us bow down to the world and pay our due to its reality. Render unto Caesar. Humor brings us down with a pratfall. Heavy meaningful reality becomes suspect, seen through, the world laughable—paranoia dissolved, as synchronicity becomes spontaneity.

Thus the relation of the soul analyst to the spiritual event is not in terms of the doctrines or of the contents. Our concern is with the person, the Who, going up the mountain. Also we ask, Who is already up there, calling?

This question is not so different from one put in spiritual disciplines, and it is crucial. For it is not the trip and its stations and path, not the rate of ascent and the rung of the ladder, or the peak and its experience, nor even the return—it is the person in the person prompting the whole endeavor. And here we fall back into history, the historical ego, our Western-Northern willpower, the very willpower that brought the missionaries and trappers, the cattlemen and ranchers and planters, the Okies and Arkies, the orange-growers, wine-growers, and sectarians, and the gold-rushers and railroaders to California to begin with. Can this be left at the door like a dusty pair of outworn shoes when one goes into the sweet-smelling pad of the meditation room? Can one close the door on the person who brought one to the threshold in the first place?

The movement from one side of the brain to the other, from tedious daily life in the supermarket to supraconsciousness, from trash to transcendence, the "altered state of conscious-ness" approach—to put it all in a nutshell—denies this historical ego. It is an approach going back to Saul who became Paul, conversion into the opposite, knocked off one's ass in a flash.

So you see the archetypal question is neither *how* does the soul/spirit conflict happen, nor *why*, but *who* among the variety of figures of which we are each composed, which archetypal figure or person, is in this happening? What God is at work in calling us up the mountain or in holding us to the vales? For archetypal psychology, there is a God in every perspective, in every position. All things are determined by psychic images, including our formulations of the spirit. All things present themselves to consciousness in the shapings of one or another divine perspective. Our vision is mimetic to one or another of the Gods.

Who is going up the mountain: is it the unconscious do-gooder Christian in us, he who has lost his historical Christianity and is an unconscious crusader, knight, missionary, savior? (I tend to see the latent "Christian Soldier" of our unconscious Christianity as more of a social danger than so-called latent psychosis, or latent homosexuality, or masked, latent depression.)

Who is going up the mountain: is it the Climber, a man who would become the mountain himself; I on Mount Rushmore—humble now, but you just wait and see. . . .

Is it the heroic ego? Is it Hercules, still at the same labors: cleaning up the stables of pollution, killing the swamp creatures, clubbing his animals, refusing the call of women, progressing through twelve stages (all in the end to go mad and marry Hebe, who is Hera, Mom, in her younger, sweeter, smilingly hebephrenic form)?

Or is the one ascending the spiritual impetus of the *puer aeternus*,[23] the winged godlike imago in us each, the beautiful boy of the spirit—Icarus on the way to the sun, then plummeting with waxen wings; Phaëthon driving the sun's chariot out of control, burning up the world; Bellerophon, ascending on his white winged horse, then falling onto the plains of wandering, limping ever after? These are the *puer* high climbers, the heaven stormers, whose eros reflects the torch and ladder of Eros and his searching arrow, a longing for higher and further and more and purer and better. Without this archetypal component affecting our lives, there would be no spiritual drive, no new sparks, no going beyond the given, no grandeur and sense of personal destiny.

So, psychologically, and perhaps spiritually as well, the issue is one of finding connections between the *puer*'s drive upward and the soul's clouded, encumbering embrace. My notion of this connection would avoid two side tracks. The first would take the soul up too, "liberate it" from its vale—the transcendentalist's demand. The second would reduce the spirit to a complex and would thus deny the *puer*'s legitimate ambition and art of flying—the psychoanalyst's demand. Let's remember here that he who cannot fly cannot imagine, as Gaston Bachelard said, and also Muhammad Ali. To imagine in a true high-flying, free-falling way, to walk on air and put on airs, to experience pneumatic reality and its concomitant inflation, one must imagine out of the valley, above the grainfields and the daily bread. Sometimes this is too much for professional analysts, and by not recognizing the archetypal claims of the *puer,* they thwart imagination.

Let us now turn to the *puer*-psyche connection without forcing the claims of either figure upon the other.

## IV. THE *PUER*-PSYCHE MARRIAGE

The accommodation between the high-driving spirit on the one hand and the nymph, the valley, or the soul on the other can be imagined as the *puer*-psyche marriage. It has been recounted in many ways—for instance, in Jung's *Mysterium Coniunctionis* as an alchemical conjunction of personified substances, or in Apuleius's tale of Eros and Psyche.[24] In the same manner as these models, let us imagine in a personified style. Then we can feel the different needs within us as volitions of distinct persons, where *puer* is the Who in our spirit flight, and anima (or psyche) is the Who in our soul.

Now the main thing about the anima[25] is just what has always been said about the psyche: it is unfathomable, ungraspable. For the anima, "the archetype of life," as Jung has called her, is that function of the psyche which is its actual life, the present mess it is in, its discontent, dishonesties, and thrilling illusions, together with the whitewashing hopes for a better outcome. The issues she presents are as endless as the soul is deep, and perhaps these very endless labyrinthine "problems" *are* its depth. The anima embroils and twists and screws us to the breaking point, performing the "function of relationship," another of Jung's definitions, a definition that becomes convincing only when we realize that relationship means perplexity.

This mess of psyche is what *puer* consciousness needs to marry so as to undertake "the battle of the sexes." The opponents of the spirit are first of all the hassles under its own skin: the morning moods, the symptoms, the prevarications in which it gets entangled, and the vanity. The *puer* needs to battle the irritability of this inner "woman," her passive laziness, her fancies for sweets and flatteries—all that which analysis calls "autoeroticism." This fighting is a fighting *with*, rather than a fighting off or fighting against, the anima, a close, tense, devoted embracing in many positions of intercourse, where *puer* madness is met with psychic confusion and deviation, and where this madness is reflected in that distorted mirror. It is not straight and not clear. We do not even know what weapons to use or where the enemy is, since the enemy seems to be my own soul and heart and most dear passions. The *puer* is left only with his craziness, which, through the battle, he has resort to so often that he learns to care for it as precious, as the one thing that he truly is, his uniqueness and limitation. Reflection in the mirror of the soul lets one see the madness of one's spiritual drive, and the importance of this madness.

Precisely this is what the struggle with the anima, and what psychotherapy as the place of this struggle, is all about: to discover one's madness, one's unique spirit, and to see the relationship between one's spirit and one's madness, that there is madness in one's spirit, and there is spirit in one's madness.

The spirit needs witness to this madness. Or to put it another way, the *puer* takes its drive and goal literally unless there is reflection, which makes possible a metaphorical understanding of its drive and goal. By bearing witness as the receptive experiencer and imager of the spirit's actions, the soul can contain, nourish, and elaborate in fantasy the *puer* impulse, bring it sensuousness and depth, involve it in life's delusions, care for it for better or for worse. Then the individual in whom these two components are marrying begins to carry with him his own reflective mirror and echo. He becomes aware of what his spiritual actions mean in terms of psyche. The spirit turned toward psyche, rather than deserting it for high places and cosmic love, finds ever further possibilities of seeing through the opacities and obfuscations in the valley. Sunlight enters the vale. The Word participates in gossip and chatter.

The spirit asks that the psyche help it, not break it or yoke it or put it away as a peculiarity or insanity. And it asks the analysts who act in psyche's name not to turn the soul against the *puer* adventure but rather to prepare the desire of both for each other.

Unfortunately a good deal of the psychotherapeutic cosmos is dominated by the perspective of Hera's social adaptation (and her favorite minion, the strong ego of coping Hercules). Hera is out to get the renegade *puer* spirit and "do" something sensible with it. The *puer* spirit is not seen for its authentic archetypal value. Hera's priests and priestesses of psychological counseling attempt to make problems clearer, give therapeutic support, by trying to understand what upsets a person. Psychological counseling then literalizes problems and, by killing the possibility of seeing through to their madness, kills the spirit.

Psychologists who do not attend enough to spirit forget that it is one of the essential components of the conjunction and cannot be dismissed as a head trip, as intellect, as just theology or metaphysics or a *puer* flight. Spirit neglected comes into psychology through the back door, disguised as synchronicity, magic, oracles, science fiction, self-symbolism, mandalas, tarot, astrology, and other indiscriminations, equally prophetic, ahistorical, and humorless. For it requires spirit to discern among the spirits.

*Diakrisis* itself is a gift of the spirit, and psychologists who refuse the *puer* chug along empowered by doctrinal mechanisms of dead masters, their own imaginative sails decayed or never even hoisted, circling in the doldrums of low-profile, low-horizon humility: the practice of psychotherapy.

Once the spirit has turned toward the soul, the soul can regard its own needs in a new way. Then these needs are no longer attempts to adapt to Hera's civilizational requirements, or to Venus's insistence that love is God, or to Apollo's medical cures, or even Psyche's work of soul-making. Not for the sake of learning love only, or for community, or for better marriages and better families, or for independence does the psyche present its symptoms and neurotic claims. Rather these demands are asking also for inspiration, for long-distance vision, for ascending eros, for vivification and intensification (*not* relaxation), for radicality, transcendence, and meaning—in short, the psyche has spiritual needs, which the *puer* part of us can fulfill. Soul asks that its preoccupations be not dismissed as trivia but seen through in terms of higher and deeper perspectives, the verticalities of the spirit. When we realize that our psychic malaise points to a spiritual hunger beyond what psychology offers and that our spiritual dryness points to a need for psychic waters beyond what spiritual discipline offers, then we are beginning to move both therapy and discipline.

The *puer*-psyche marriage results first of all in increased interiority. It constructs a walled space, the thalamus or bridal chamber, neither peak nor vale, but rather a place where both can be looked at through glass windows or be closed off with doors. This increased interiority means that each new *puer* inspiration, each hot idea, at whatever time of life in whomever, be given psychization. It will first be drawn through the labyrinthine ways of the soul, which wind it and slow it and nourish it from many sides (the "many" nurses and "many" maenads), developing the spirit from a one-way mania for "ups" to *polytropos*, the many-sidedness of the Hermetic old hero, Ulysses. The soul performs the service of indirection to the *puer* arrow, bringing to the sulphuric compulsions of the spirit the lasting salt of soul.

Likewise, for soul: the bridal chamber intensifies the brooding, gives it heat and pressure, building soul from amorphous clouds into driving needs. And these, by benefit of *puer*, become formulated into language. There is a sense of process, direction, continuity within one's interior life of dreams and wishes. Suffering begins to make sense. Instead of the repetitious and usual youth-nymph pairings of virginal innocence coupled with seed spilled everywhere foolishly, psychic conception takes place and the opus of one's life begins to form.

The *puer*-psyche marriage finally implies taking our complexes both out of the world and out of the realm of spiritual systems. It means that the search and questing go through a psychological search and questing, an exploration of soul by spirit for psychic fecundation. The messianic, liberating, transcending movement connects first with soul and is concerned first with its movement: not "what does this mean?"—the question asked of spirit by spirit—but "what does this move in my soul?"—the interiorization of the question. This alone puts psychic body into the *puer* message and trip, adding to it psychic values, so that the *puer* message can touch soul and redden it into life. For it is especially in this realm of soul—so lost, emptied, and ignorant—that the gifts of the *puer* spirit are first needed. It is soul, psyche, and psychology that need the spirit's attention. Come down from the mountain, monks, and like beautiful John Keats, come into the vale of soul-making.

## V. FOUR POINTS OF DIFFERENCE

At this point I am leaving the *puer*'s enthusiastic perspective to return again to soul. I want to suggest now three fundamental qualities of soul-making in distinction to spirit disciplines. These three are: (1) *Pathologizing*[26]—an interest in the psycho-pathologies of our lives—that is, an attentive concern to the logos of the pathos of the psyche. By keeping an ear tuned to the soul's pathologizings, we maintain the close link of soul with mortality, limitation, and death. (2) *Anima*—a loyalty to the clouded moods at the water sources, to the seductive twists and turns of the interior feminine figures who personify the labyrinthine path of psychic life, those nymphs, dark witches, lost cinderellas, and persephones of destruction, and the elusive, illusional fantasies that anima creates, the images of soul in the soul. (3) *Polytheism*—single-minded commitment to discord and cacophony, to variety and not getting it all together, to falling apart, the multiplicity of the ten thousand things, to the peripheries and their tangents (rather than centers), to the episodic, occasional, wandering movement of the soul (like this lecture) and its compulsion to repeat in the valleys of its errors, and the necessity of errancy and error for discovering the many ways of many Gods.

I am aware that these lectures have been organized in order to relate East and West, religious disciplines and psychotherapy, and so I must make a contribution to an issue that I believe is not the main one (the East-West pair). For I believe the true passion is between North and South, between the upper and lower regions, whether they be the repressive Northern Protestantism of Europe and America on the one hand, and on the other, Southland, the oppressed Mediterranean, the Latin darkness below the borders, across the rivers, under the alps; whether this division be the manic industrial North and the depressive ritualistic South, or between San Francisco and Los Angeles.

But Professor Needleman says the line is blurred between the therapist and the spiritual guide, and he would draw that line spiritually—that is, vertically—creating East and West across the mountaintops, perhaps like the Continental Divide, whereas I would draw the line horizontally, as rivers flow, downward. The three qualifications I have just made—pathologizing, anima, polytheism—are my way of drawing the line more heavily and bluntly, thick with shadow.

Anyone who is engaged with these three factors, regarding them as important, as religious even, seems to me to be engaged in therapy and psychology. Anyone who tends to dismiss pathologizing for growth, or anima confusions for ego strength or spiritual illumination, or who neglects the differentiation of multiplicity and variety for the sake of unity is engaged in spiritual discipline.

The lines between the two labors I would draw in this way. But I would also suggest that they are drawn not by what a person preaches but according to the weight of importance he lays upon trivia, the little things in daily practice. There are, for instance, many who are called psychotherapists and pretend its practice, but who, according to these criteria, are actually daily engaged in spirit. In the emphasis they give and in the values they select, their main concern is with ascension (growing *up*), strengthening, unity, and wholeness. Whereas I believe, though I am less familiar with the spiritual side of things (coming from Switzerland, where our main words are *complex, schizophrenia, introvert-extrovert, Rorschach* and *Bleuler,* and the spectrum of drugs from Ciba-Geigy, Sandoz, and Hoffmann–La Roche; that is, our fantasy is more psychiatric, more psychopathological than yours, which is more spiritually determined by your history and geography, this Golden State, its founding missions, its holy spiritual names— Eureka, Sacramento, Berkeley [the Bishop], Los Angeles, San Diego, Santa Cruz, Carmel, Santa Barbara) I believe that the spiritual masters may, despite their doctrine, very often be engaged in psychotherapy when they follow the female inner figure as guide, the *paredros* or angel, when they allow vision and fantasy to flourish, when they let the multiple voices in the symptoms speak and turn the pathologizings into inner teachers, when they move from all generalities and abstractions to concrete immediacy and the multivalence of events.

In other words, the lines between therapy and discipline, between soul and spirit, do not depend on the kind of patient, or the kind of teacher, or whether the patient or teacher was born in the Cascades or the Himalayas, but rather depend upon which archetypal dominant is working through one's viewpoint. The issue always returns to "Who" in an individual's subjectivity is asking the questions and giving the answers.

Pathologizing, anima, and polytheism are, moreover, intimately connected with one another. It would take us too far in this talk to attempt to show the internal logic of this connection, and I am not up to doing it swiftly and succinctly. Besides, this interconnection has been a main theme of many of my writings, because one soon discovers in work with oneself and others that each of these criteria of soul-making tends to imply the other. The varied anima figures, elfin inspirations, and moods that move a person, men and women alike (for it is nonsense to hold that women can have only animuses, no souls, as if an archetype or a goddess could be limited to the personal psychology of sexual gender), give a peculiar double feeling. There is a sense of me-ness, personal importance, soul sense, that is not an ego inflation, and at the same time there is an awareness of one's subjectivity being fluid, airy, fiery, earthy, made of many components, shifting, ungraspable, now close and intimate and helpful as Athena giving wise counsel, then wily and disappearing, naïvely pulling one into hopeless holes like Persephone, and at the next moment fantasizing Aphroditic whisperings in the inner ear, sea foam, pink vulvar bivalves, and then proud and tall Artemis, keeping everything at bay, oneself at a distance, at one only with nature, a virgin soul among brothers and sisters, only.

Anima makes us feel many parts.

Anima, as Jung said, is an equivalent of and a personfication of the polytheistic aspect of the psyche.[27] "Polytheism" is a theological or anthropological concept for the experience of a many-souled world.

This same experience of multiplicity can reach us as well through symptoms. They too make us aware that the soul has other voices and intentions than the one of the ego. Pathologizing bears witness to both the soul's inherent composite nature and to the many Gods reflected in this composition. Here I take my cue from two passing remarks of Jung. "The divine thing in us functions as neuroses of the stomach, or the colon, or the bladder, simply disturbances of the underworld. Our Gods have gone to sleep, and they only stir in the bowels of the earth." [28] And again: "The gods have become diseases; Zeus no longer rules Olympus but rather the solar plexus, and produces curious specimens for the doctor's consulting room. . . ." [29]

Sometimes going up the mountain one seeks escape from this underworld, and so the Gods appear from below bringing all sorts of physiological disorders. They will be heard, if only through intestinal rumblings and their fire burning in the bladder.

Like going up the mountain, but in the disguise of psychology, are the behavior therapies and release-relax therapies. Cure the symptom and lose the God. Had Jacob not grappled with the Daemon he would indeed have not been hurt, and he would not have been Jacob either. Lose the symptom and return the world back to the ego.

Here my point is that soul-making does not deny Gods and the search for them. But it looks closer to hand, finding them more in the manner of the Greeks and Egyptians, for whom the Gods take part in all things. All existence is filled with them, and human beings are always involved with them. This involvement is what myths are all about—the traditional stories of human and divine interactions. There is no place one can be, no act one can do, no thought one can think without it being mimetic to a God. Thus we study mythology to understand personality structure, psychodynamics, pathologizing. The Gods are within, as Heinrich Zimmer used to say, and they are within our acts, thoughts, and feelings. We do not have to trek across the starry spaces to them, the brain of heaven, or blast them loose from concealment with mind-blowing chemicals. They are there in the very ways you feel and think and experience your moods and symptoms. Here is Apollo, right here, making us distant and wanting to form artful, clear, and distinct ideas; here is old Saturn, imprisoned in paranoid systems of judgment, defensive maneuvers, melancholic conclusions; here is Mars, having to turn red in the face and kill in order to make a point; and here too is the wood nymph Daphne-Diana, retreating into foliage, the camouflage of innocence, suicide through naturalness.

Finally, I would point to one more, a fourth, difference between peaks and vales, the difference that has to do with death.

If spirit would transcend death in any of several ways—unification so that one is not subject to dissolution; union with self, where self is God; building the immortal body, or the jade-body; the moves toward timelessness and spacelessness and imagelessness and mindlessness; dying to the world as place of attachments—soul-making would instead hew and bevel the ship of death, the vessel of death, a container for holding the dying that goes on in the soul. It imagines that psychic life refers most fundamentally to the life of the *po*-soul, that which slips into the ground—not just at the moment of physical death but is always slipping into the ground, always descending, always going deeper into concrete realities and animating them.

So I cannot conclude with ultimates, positions, final words, wise statements from masters. There is no end to a wandering discourse, no summation, summit, for to make an end is to come to a stop. I'd rather leave unconcluded and cloudy, no abstracted spiritual message—not even a particular image. You have your own. The soul generates them ceaselessly.

# Notes

1. C. J. Hefele, *Conciliengeschichte* (Freiburg i/Breisgau: Herder, 1860), IV: 320, 404 (Canon 11).
2. D. L. Miller, "Achelous and the Butterfly," *Spring 1973* (New York/Zurich: Spring Publications), p. 14.

3. Cf. M. T. Kelsey, *God, Dreams, and Revelation* (Minneapolis: Augsburg Publishing House, 1974), pp. 80–84; A. N. Wilder, "Myth and Dream in Christian Scripture," in *Myths, Dreams and Religion*, ed. J. Campbell (New York: Dutton, 1970), pp. 68–75; H. Schar, *"Bemerkungen zu Träumen der Bibel,"* in *Traum und Symbol* (Zürich: Rascher, 1963), pp. 171–79.

4. C. G. Hefele, *A History of the Councils of the Church*, transl. W. R. Clark (Edinburgh: Clark, 1896), V: 260–400, esp. pp. 377–85.

5. Hefele, *Conciliengeschichte*, IV: 402 (Canon 3).

6. C. G. Jung, *Collected Works* (Princeton University Press, Bollingen Series), VIII: para. 92.

7. Jung, *Collected Works*, VI: para. 66, 77.

8. Jung, *Collected Works*, VIII: para. 618, 623; XI: para. 769.

9. Jung, *Collected Works*, VIII: para. 746.

10. Jung, *Collected Works*, XI: para. 889.

11. Jung, *Collected Works*, VI: para. 743.

12. Jung, *Collected Works*, VI: para. 78.

13. W. H. Roscher, *Ausführliches Lexikon der griechischen und römischen Mythologie* (Leipzig/Stuttgart: Teubner; Hildesheim: Olms, 1965), "Pan," pp. 1392 f.

14. V. MacDermott, *The Cult of the Seer in the Ancient Middle East* (Berkeley/Los Angeles: University of California Press, 1971). Cf. H. Frankfort, *Ancient Egyptian Religion* (New York: Harper Torchbook, 1961), Chapter 1, for an excellent summary of Egyptian polytheistic psychology.

15. MacDermott, p. 46.

16. E. M. Forster, *Aspects of the Novel* (1927) (Harmondsworth: Pelican, 1971), p. 115.

17. Forster, p. 115.

18. Forster, p. 129.

19. Forster, p. 116.

20. Forster, p. 116.

21. On the relation of humor and psyche, see Miller, pp. 1–23.

22. On synchronicity and Pan, see my "An Essay on Pan" in *Pan and the Nightmare* (with W. H. Roscher) (New York/Zurich: Spring Publications, 1972), pp. lvi–lix.

23. Cf. M.-L. von Franz, *The Problem of the Puer Aeternus* (New York/Zurich: Spring Publications, 1970), and my several papers on the theme—e.g., "Pothos—The Nostalgia of the Puer Aeternus" in *Loose Ends: Primary Papers in Archetypal Psychology* (New York/Zurich: Spring Publications, 1974), pp. 49–62.

24. There are many Jungian interpretative attempts on this tale. Cf. M.-L.

von Franz, *A Psychological Interpretation of the Golden Ass of Apuleius* (New York/Zurich, 1970); E. Neumann, *Amor and Psyche* (New York: Pantheon, 1956); and my own *The Myth of Analysis* (Evanston: Northwestern University Press, 1972), pp. 55 ff.

25. For a full exploration of anima, relevant literature, and citations from Jung, see my two papers "Anima" in *Spring 1973*, pp. 97–132, and *1974*, pp. 113–46.

26. By *pathologizing* I mean the psyche's autonomous ability to create illness, morbidity, disorder, abnormality, and suffering in any aspect of its behavior and to experience and imagine life through this deformed and afflicted perspective; cf. "Pathologizing," part two of my *Re-Visioning Psychology* (New York: Harper & Row, 1975).

27. Jung, *Collected Works*, IX, ii: para 427 and my discussion of this theme in "Psychology: Monotheistic or Polytheistic?," *Spring 1971*, pp. 193–208.

28. C. G. Jung, "Psychological Commentary on Kundalini Yoga" (from the Notes of Mary Foote, 1932), *Spring 1975*, p. 22.

29. Jung, *Collected Works*, XIII: para. 54.

# James Hillman: *Questions*

*Question:* What's the proper response of the spiritual discipline to what the soul generates?

*Dr. Hillman:* Now I don't know what it *does*, but I do know what would be damaging, what would prevent the marriage of spirit and soul. Let's take a moment of meditation when you are supposed to focus upon something—whatever it is, whether it's to empty yourself out, or focus upon a particular image or thought or sentence. Then something invades your mind: you know, some absurd thing, some TV ad you saw the day before, or whatever. Now, from the psychological point of view, that's the psyche speaking; and one concentrates on what *appears*, one follows *it*, listens to *it*, rather than trying to suppress it by concentrating on what has been prescribed. That's an essential aspect in Jung's notion of active imagination. So the proper response would be: accepting what comes, whatever comes, and working with that.

*Question:* There's a phrase that is supposedly used by old people sometimes in talking of youth and they say, "Youth, it's such a pity that it's wasted on the young." Old people have never said it to me—they've been kind. But as people grow older and look back on their lives and see they've lived a good deal of it in the valleys, is it any wonder that they wish for something different, perhaps to be on the peaks? You seem to think that that wish is perhaps naïve—not wrong, but naïve.

*Answer:* Well, first of all, "naïve" is one of the words used about the *puer*, and it depends on what one does with that "naïve." I don't necessarily see that term as a condemnation. Whatever *begins* is naïve. Beginnings are naïve, you know. I think the mistake here is in talking about old people and young

142

people, rather than of two archetypes—of *puer* and *senex*. And one can have the *senex* at any age, and one can have the *puer* in one at any age. T. S. Eliot says: "Old men ought to be explorers," because for them "here and there does not matter."

*Question:* Yes, but the old do not have the physical vitality that enables them to be explorers. They sit back and they see young people doing the same things they did when they were young—in essence wasting their time when they could be exploring. And I think that is the source of that phrase—that youth is wasted on the young.

*Answer:* I don't know whether you've got the thing concretized too much there, in the sense of physical vitality in particular age groups. One can be an "old man" at any age. And one can be a *puer*—or one can *have* the *puer* spark at any age. What makes the so-called "wise old man" so foolish, spontaneous, childlike, irrational, able to fall in love again? That is the moment of the *puer*. The *puer* archetype can as easily work in a person who is seventy as in a person who is twenty. I think we have to free these notions from their location in a particular age group.

*Question:* You said that you don't want to deny women's soul—deny the anima for women. Do you feel that the *puer* archetype can be used for women's spirit, just as it can for men?

*Answer:* Certainly. Let's use the word *Gods* and drop *archetypes* for a moment. You can be a man or a woman and be *informed* by Athena or Zeus or Hermes; it doesn't matter whether you're a man or a woman. The *puer aeternus*—the soaring, the ascension, the fire, the wings, the inspiration, the longing—a whole series of phenomena—and the woundedness, and the interest in destruction, and so forth, can also appear in women's psychology. I don't think the Gods are limited by the personal gender of gender.

*Question:* Would you connect the *puer* aspect with the animus—with Jung's notion of the animus?

*Answer:* I think animus and anima are again both persons and abstractions. It depends on how we use these terms. If we take animus as a general concept, then we can have all sorts of animuses—all sorts of images—sailors and teachers and judges and the various Gods and so on. But certainly one aspect of the traditional notion of animus is *puer,* which is fascinating to a woman. It leads her into spirit and all the same sorts of foolishnesses that we men are led into.

*Question:* What about efforts to push the pathology to see what it may bring out in us. In the middle of, say, attacking your mate or difficulties you're in, you feel free to go on to see even how far it can go. To see what will happen to me, what may come out of me, what may come.

*Answer:* Yes. Absolutely. I think that's very important: to be able to listen to it, I mean give it the time. Because it invades and demands the time.

*Question:* What was the question?

*Answer:* The question was "Should one push one's pathologies?"

*Question:* [But that wasn't all of the question. He said something about attacking his mate.]

*Answer:* I thought he said *rather* than attacking his mate. [Laughter.] The attack on the mate, the battle of the sexes—that was a metaphor. And I thought that you were saying the same thing—the internal mate. The moods, the symptoms.

*Question:* Right.

*Answer:* Right. Listening to them. Fighting with them in different ways, getting involved with them.

*Question:* Okay. But if those moods then involve relationships with other people to the point of pushing yourself against them, changing your environment, fighting other people—do we go along with that?

*Answer:* Well, wouldn't you say that you're not giving the moods attention so that they then demand that attention from other people? See, it's the question of personifying or objectifying. That's why I speak of a "mate." There it is, it's with you all day long, you know? I mean, you can't even leave it at home when you go out. That thing, if you don't take care of it, it begins to make all sorts of demands elsewhere. It starts looking around.

*Question:* What about the parts in us that are destructive?

*Answer:* Well, now we're into something else. Now we're into this question of the parts of us that are declared destructive. Who's the judge here? Who's the prosecuting attorney? Who's deciding who's destructive?

*Question:* I decide when I think that I may be destroying somebody else's life—not in the physical sense of killing, but detracting from them. And then I say, "Okay. Stop or change or look and do something different."

*Answer:* But everything you've said so far has stayed with this "I." You haven't let the thing that's doing it say what it wants.

Now we're into the question of personifying the complexes. This is an essential part of recognizing oneself as a multitude of persons or as a multiple person, so that one cannot decide the whole thing as the sergeant—oneself for the whole platoon—but must let the other people say something. Regarding oneself as a commune of voices, with faces. This is what I meant by a multiple or diverse or polytheistic approach to the psyche.

*Question:* Then could you take the notion of suicide and ask whether that means that you go out and kill yourself? What are the other options when you have images in the psyche of suicide?

*Answer:* Well, again, the problem is one of literalizing, or what has been called classically in psychoanalysis as "acting out." Everything that the psyche presents is metaphorical. If you have images of suicide, there is some kind of movement toward the realm of death. It's an attempt to get to death in one way or another, or to leave some kind of thing that has been identified with as life. Whether it's body or world or family, or something of that sort. Don't you think that each one of these so-called destructive things is a statement of some kind? I'm not saying there isn't destruction—it's just that one has to *listen* to it first.

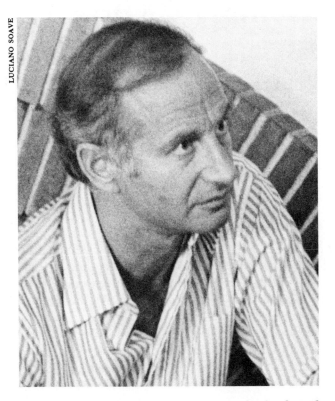

*James Hillman,* Dr. Phil., is American by birth and Swiss by residence, with degrees from the Sorbonne, Trinity College Dublin, and the University of Zurich. He was Director of Studies at the C. G. Jung Institute in Zurich for ten years and participates regularly at the Eranos Conferences at Ascona. His published works include *Insearch—Psychology and Religion, The Myth of Analysis* and *Revisioning Psychology.*

# DRUGS, YOGA, AND PSYCHOTRANSFORMISM

## Robert S. de Ropp

"Drugs, Yoga, and Psychotransformism": when I read this title to the group of people who work with me, they shrieked with laughter, which is the kind of irreverent response I've become accustomed to. "Psychotransformism" was what triggered this outburst of merriment.

*Transformism*, of course, originally referred to the theory that living things were not created by an act of God but by the gradual transformation of one form into another. This theory was later stated by Darwin and Wallace as the Theory of Evolution.

*Psychotransformism* was a word used by P. D. Ouspensky to describe a series of changes that can take place in the psyche of man. Psychotransformism deals with the possibility of man transforming himself from a being who is Public Enemy #1 from the point of view of the biosphere—a very disharmonized, dangerous creature—to a being who can live in harmony with both himself and the universe. According to this theory man has in himself possibilities for development that he generally does not even know about, let alone use. Nature guarantees that man will develop up to the stage of a sexually mature animal. At this point she leaves him to his own devices. Whether he develops further or not depends entirely on his own desires. He may, and generally does, live like a fool and die like a dog, in which case he becomes merely "food for worms." Or he may, through certain kinds of intentional effort, transform himself into a higher kind of being, in which case he is incorporated into an upward-moving part of the cosmic process.

The theory of psychotransformism is such that anyone can test its validity. Anyone can test it because man can always use himself as his own guinea pig to see if it works. There is nothing to believe, only an experiment to be undertaken.

In order to study this theory scientifically it is necessary to consider the structure and function of the human brain. The brain of man is the most complex and dangerous of all the devices that have developed on earth's biosphere. It is a horrendously disharmonized organ. Its disharmony results from the fact that it is not one but many. It incorporates three different brains in a single entity: an instinctive brain about on the level of a crocodile, an emotional brain not much above the level of that of a horse, and perched on top of this highly unstable combination like a king on a very wobbly throne, a recently evolved man-brain, housed in two enormously overdeveloped cerebral hemispheres.

Now it stands to reason that any being who is unfortunate enough to have to create some sort of harmony between a crocodile, horse, and man is going to have some difficulty. One has only to read human history to see what a ghastly mess this mixture has made. Arthur Koestler, in *The Ghost in the Machine*, has suggested that man is a victim of an error in brain formation. The error resulted from the failure of the old brain to evolve harmoniously with the new brain. The result was a biological disaster, which may lead not only to the extinction of the human race itself but to irreparable damage to the biosphere of the planet earth.

So the burning question, compared with which all other questions are trivial, is this: does the human brain have in itself the capacity first to recognize its own defects and second to remedy these defects?

FIGURE 1

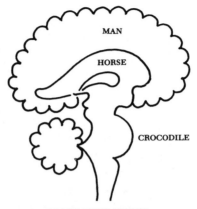

BRAIN HIERARCHY

The theory of psychotransformism answers that man's position is difficult and dangerous but not hopeless. The brain, like certain highly sophisticated computers, has the ability to recognize and correct some of its errors. To do this, however, it must use a brain system that, though it certainly exists in man, is not generally recognized. It lies unused like a powerful machine that its owner does not even know he possesses.

If we look at the brain systems that determine the behavior of men and the other animals, we see that two systems predominate. Following John Lilly we will call them the stop system and the start system. The two systems are intimately associated with reward and punishment. The start system offers the animal its rewards. It is more or less synonymous with the pleasure center, the power of which was demonstrated so dramatically by Olds in the rat and Lilly in the monkey. Implant an electrode in the pleasure center of a rat or a monkey and hook it up to a bar the creature can press and you will have a fascinating, even frightening demonstration of the power this center can exert. Hour after hour, neglecting all its other needs, the animal will sit there pressing the bar. It is literally a slave to its pleasure center.

FIGURE 2

## PSYCHODYNAMICS

## BRAIN SYSTEMS

| ✿ | ✿ |
| --- | --- |
| START | STOP |
| ACTION | INACTION |
| PLEASURE | PAIN |
| REWARDS | PUNISHMENT |

NEUROHORMONES

| | |
| --- | --- |
| NOREPINEPHRINE | ACETYLCHOLINE |

The effect of the stop system is equally dramatic, though fortunately for us it is located in a very small part of the brain. This brain system punishes the animal so drastically that if an electrode implanted there is activated frequently the creature goes into a decline, loses interest in life, and finally dies. The only way to halt its decline is to activate the start system.

It is worth noting that these two systems depend for their functioning on two different chemicals. The pleasure, or start, system depends on the neurohormone norepinephrine; the pain, or stop, system depends on the neurohormone acetylcholine. It is very important that we realize how totally our moods and our whole sense of what we call "self" depend on minute traces of certain chemicals, the neurohormones, liberated at the ends of our nerve fibers. A defect in the metabolism of norepinephrine can plunge a person into the depths of a totally inexplicable depression or induce the hallucinations of schizophrenia. The medical men will shake their heads, and if they are psychoanalytically inclined will pass the patient on to a psychiatric colleague, who will put the person through the ropes, charging fifty dollars an hour. But this is useless, because the real problem is one of chemistry. All forms of behavior can ultimately be traced to events at the molecular level occurring in certain areas of the brain. The so-called psychotropic drugs act on the brain by affecting these biochemical processes.

The stop and start systems underlie all ordinary human behavior. Man seeks for stimuli that will activate the pleasure center. With equal earnestness he seeks to avoid any influences that will activate the pain center. He moves like a donkey between the stick and the carrot, a blundering beast driven by impulses he can hardly understand on a journey that has no real aim and makes no real sense. Whether chasing after pleasure or running away from pain, he is a slave to those tyrannical brain centers, the stop and start systems, which limit his freedom and turn him into a helpless puppet.

*"Filthy old nature, she drives us amain.*
*The one goad is lust and the other is pain."*

These words, shouted by a madman in one of H. G. Wells's more inspired novels, summarizes man's condition at the level of being on which he usually exists. But the theory of psychotransformism states that he does not have to exist on this wretched level. Man's new brain, the neocortex, is a large, complex, and truly magnificent organ, which its possessor does not know how to use. It is like an extraordinary computer placed in the hands of an ignorant peasant who hasn't the foggiest idea what it is for. And, even worse, the instruction book has been lost.

In addition to the stop and start centers, which man shares with other animals, the neocortex contains higher centers, the centers of power and of liberation. He who can activate these centers ceases to be a slave of the pleasure-pain dyad. Such a person attains a certain inner freedom coupled with a totally new understanding of himself and his power—he has fulfilled his potential and become truly a man.

The theory of psychotransformism states that although these higher centers exist in the brain of man, they can be activated only through intentional efforts. It is as if nature presented man with a superb gift and later, repenting of her generosity, placed in his psyche certain obstacles that would make it almost impossible for him to use the gift. In the New Testament, which is a treatise on psychotransformism written in code, we find this idea referred to in several parables. The higher center in man's brain offers the keys to that state called the "kingdom of heaven." Man does not ordinarily know that the kingdom exists. If he belongs to the so-called Christian Church, he may have been told that it exists somewhere in the stratosphere and is peopled with improbable fauna-like cherubs and angels or that it is some state only attained after death. But the kingdom of heaven exists in his own brain. It is up to him to find it. So in the New Testament parable the kingdom of heaven is compared to treasure hidden in a field, which, when a man discovered it, he went and sold all that he possessed and bought the field.

The same idea is presented somewhat differently in the parable of the prodigal son. The prodigal son, having squandered his substance on riotous living, finds himself reduced to the level of a swineherd who "would fain fill his belly with the husks which the swine did eat." Only in this dire extremity does he remember his father's house and resolve at all costs to return there.

These parables express allegorically two of the most important principles of psychotransformism. First, before man can even begin to develop, he must realize that as long as he remains a slave to the pleasure and pain centers his life is no better than that of an animal. He is a swine among swine. In fact he is lower than they are because at least they have no higher potential to throw away. Second, he must understand that to enter the kingdom of heaven in the Gospel allegory he must be willing to sacrifice all that he possesses. Nature has made no provision to ensure that man will develop his full power. We can understand this by comparing man to an insect like a butterfly that passes through several forms: egg, caterpillar, chrysalis, and winged adult. Nature ensures that the insect will pass through all these stages. But man, whose ultimate inner transformation can be compared to the change from a caterpillar to a butterfly, is forced to rely entirely on his own intentional efforts to bring about this metamorphosis. Nature not only fails to help him but also places great obstacles in his way. If he wants to attain his full development and awaken the higher centers in his brain, he must work against nature. More correctly we can say he must work against nature at one level in order to serve her purposes at a higher level, for reason compels us to perceive several levels in the workings of the cosmos. Processes taking place at one level may be opposed to those taking place at another. There is no need to go as far as those Babylonian dualists and postulate two principles, a force of darkness and a force of light. It suffices to say that the process we call nature operates at several levels and that man is placed between two levels of this cosmic process. He has the possibility of transcending himself and attaining a higher level of being, or he can remain as he is, a swine among swine.

Psychotransformism deals with the laws governing self-transcendence. In many systems of teaching the process of psychotransformism is compared to a journey. This inner journey is referred to as the Way, and various levels of development are spoken of as stages of the Way. We can draw a large-scale map of the Way and distinguish five stages, as shown in Figure 3.

At the lowest level is the jungle, or treadmill, represented here as a circle, because no one at this level ever gets anywhere. People move round and round like donkeys on a treadmill. They live between the carrot and the stick. They are dragged forward by desires, desires for wealth, fame, sexual pleasure, or they are driven by fears, fear of poverty, illness, unemployment. This level is called the jungle because people in it live under the law of the jungle: eat and be eaten.

Beyond the jungle lies the forest. The forest is a better place

FIGURE 3

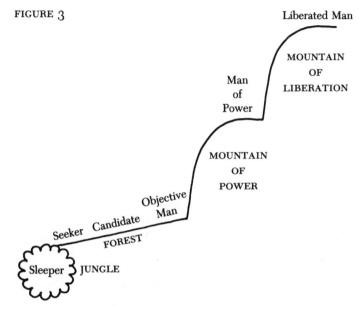

FIVE STAGES OF THE WAY

to be than the jungle. At least there are paths in the forest and some of those paths lead somewhere. There are also guides in the forest, some of whom know their way around.

The first step on the Way is to pass from the jungle into the forest. This happens when someone wakes up to the fact that life on the treadmill between the stick and the carrot is not a particularly rewarding form of existence. Such a person will start looking for a more meaningful life game. The search at this stage consists of reading books, talking to others, gathering material about the Way. All this material will form a definite entity in the seeker's persona, an entity which is called, in the system of knowledge I am describing, the magnetic center.

The seeker entering the forest has only his magnetic center to guide him. Magnetic centers can be strong and clever or weak and stupid. The function of the magnetic center is to bring the seeker in touch with a guide. Every seeker gets the guide he deserves. A fool gets a fool for a guide, a fraud gets a fraud. A person with discrimination will go on seeking until he finds a genuine guide. This is not easy. The frauds are very numerous, the genuine guides are few.

When the seeker finds his guide he begins a more intensive phase of inner work. He becomes a candidate for initiation. In the candidate the magnetic center slowly changes into a new and much more powerful entity. This entity is called the observer or the witness. At this stage the seeker has one great obligation: to see himself as he really is. Without this nothing is possible.

The seeker will see, first of all, that he has no control over his life, that he is held in this morass, this jungle, by certain functions which are symbolized in the tarot cards by the Fool, the Devil, and the Wheel of Fortune.

The Fool stands for the suggestibility and credulity in man. He'll swallow any old tale. Wandering about with his head in the air, he is about to fall over a cliff but doesn't notice it because he is immersed in dreams. He carries the four sacred symbols on his back without knowing what any of them mean—he doesn't even know why he is carrying them.

The Devil is all the lies we live in, the lies we tell ourselves and are told by our leaders.

And the Wheel of Fortune is the tendency in man to engage in totally undirected, random activity. Man does not know what he is doing. He acts on impulse, without real intention, and each impulse calls itself "I."

In order to understand the role of the observer we must realize that in his usual state of consciousness man has many selves. Each of these selves can become dominant for a time. Some of these selves are directly opposed to others. This accounts for the state of inner disharmony so characteristic of man's life in the jungle.

The function of the observer is to study these selves. He is like a manager newly appointed to take over a business that is falling apart because of failure on the part of the staff to work together. The observer studies the different selves objectively. He must decide which selves are valuable and which are dangerous. He has very little authority to begin with and cannot exercise control. Moreover he lacks objectivity and may deceive himself by refusing to see certain selves or to evaluate them correctly. Here he especially needs help from his guide.

As the observer grows in power he gradually passes out of the persona and into the essence. The persona is shallow, the essence is deep. Once the essence is reached the candidate's level of being changes. At a certain point he is no longer a candidate for initiation. He becomes an initiate of the first order. He has reached the level of objective man.

On our map of the Way we locate objective man at the foot of the first mountain, the mountain of power. Objective man has passed certain tests, the chief of which is called the undressing of the false ego. The chief characteristic of objective man is that you can neither flatter him nor insult him. He is beyond the reach of praise and blame. He has got rid of his self-importance and realized his nothingness.

It is no small thing to become objective man. Years of effort are needed plus the help of a good guide. Indeed, it may take so long for a person to reach this level that old age, the last enemy of the man of knowledge, may make any further development impossible. But if he is not too old the first-order initiate can embark on the next stage of the Way, the ascent of the mountain of power.

We now turn to a different map of the inner world of man. The mandala shown in Figure 4 is one of a class of diagrams called *yantras* and contains a great deal of information. Some of it applies to the world in which man lives, some to the inner world of man.

The large black circle around the outside is the barrier that prevents people from even beginning the great work, the great alchemical process. Then there are the three successive circles, which in the Tibetan mandala would be the circle of flames, the circle of thunderbolts, or dorjes, and the circle of lotuses.

FIGURE 4

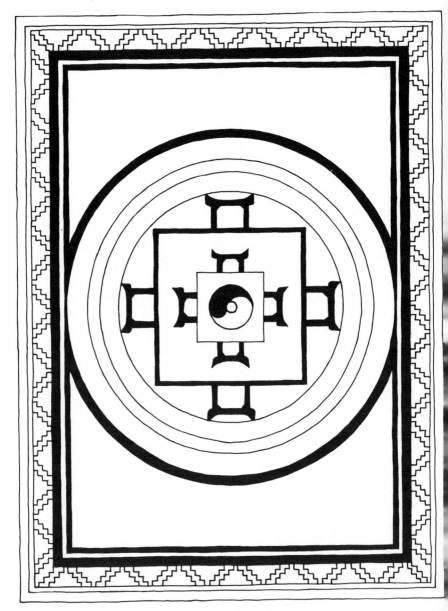

These correspond to certain energies in man which he can learn to awaken and use for inner transmutation.

The two inner squares of the mandala represent the locked rooms in the human psyche. They are equivalent to the mountain of power and the mountain of liberation shown in Figure 3. The inner chambers are approached by four gates and each gate has its guardian. Objective man, though a first-order initiate, is only on the threshold of the first square. He is in the gateway. To enter the first room he must overcome the guardian at the gate. The guardian represents certain fixed patterns of thinking, feeling, and perceiving, which hold the traveler in his familiar world. The world within the mandala is not familiar. It is, to borrow a phrase from Carlos Castaneda, "a separate reality." In the struggle to enter this strange world the traveler on the Way will encounter peculiar deceptive phenomena, the phenomena of the threshold. They have been well described by Ouspensky in *The New Model of the Universe* in a chapter entitled "Experimental Mysticism." The threshold phenomena are always products of the traveler's imagination and, however fascinating they may appear, he must dismiss them.

He who ascends the mountain of power will develop the powers, or Siddhis. One who possesses these powers can exert an influence on his fellow men. He can bend them to his will, dominate them, hypnotize them, even destroy them. He can do this because he now has unified will attained through a process called *the struggle between yes and no*. In the course of this struggle the conflicting selves in man's being are fused into a single powerful entity, an inner master. He who has created in himself this entity is a man of power, or second-order initiate.

A person can reach this stage of the Way without becoming objective man. There are certain shortcuts to the mountain of power. One who takes these shortcuts does so at his peril. He enters the sacred enclosure of the mandala still wearing his personal ego, and he will be tempted to use his powers for selfish, often destructive ends. The idea of the evil sorcerer or the black magician refers essentially to one who has taken the shortcut to the mountain of power. Among primitive peoples the shaman or witch doctor is frequently one who has taken this shortcut. Such a one is often more feared for his power to destroy than he is revered for his power to heal.

The innermost square of the mandala corresponds to the mountain of liberation in Figure 3. It is the holy of holies of man's inner temple. To this stage of the Way there are no shortcuts. One who has attained this level of being is an initiate of the third order, a perfect man, a buddha, a liberated one. It is quite impossible for such a one to misuse his powers, because he has completely transcended his personal ego. He has shed his separate consciousness and blended with the universal consciousness. He is quite unattached, does not cling to anything. To quote from the Bhagavad Gita, "He sees the Self in everything and everything in the Self." In him the process of psychotransformism has reached the ultimate stage.

At the very center of the mandala is a white spot, which is the seed of the nonmanifest world, the source of all life. The mandala as a whole represents the cosmic process of the unmanifest flowing out into the manifest through the yin-yang dyad.

Actually, the same idea is contained in a good prayer rug. The prayer rug shown in Figure 5 is based on the idea of the "inner temple" of man, the locked rooms in his psyche corresponding to the mountains of power and liberation.° Anyone who knows how to pray can enter these rooms.

I will now pass to the second theme of this talk, namely yoga. I will use the word in a very general way. The aim of all forms of yoga is the attainment of liberation from the personal ego, the source of our suffering and our illusions. Yoga underlies the spiritual practices of all the world's great

---

° It's very hard to get a good prayer rug. The people who make prayer rugs and the people who use or understand them never seem to get together and exchange ideas. You often have to make your own rug, which is what I did.

FIGURE 5

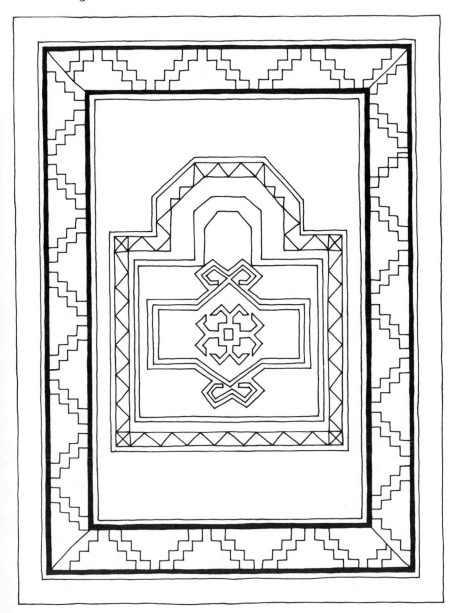

religions. There is Hindu yoga, Buddhist yoga, Christian yoga, Islamic yoga, and Taoist yoga. There are also forms of yoga quite independent of any religion. The various forms of yoga are all manifestations of three basic urges in man, which show themselves as the three higher wills: the will to power, the will to meaning, and the will to self-transcendence. Through yoga a person learns how to train these wills and to use his powers for the attainment of liberation.

The techniques of different forms of yoga relate to the natural divisions of man's being. We will consider these forms separately.

FIGURE 6

| | |
|---|---|
| HATHA YOGA | PHYSICAL BODY |
| JNANA YOGA | INTELLECT |
| BHAKTI YOGA | RELIGIOUS EMOTION |
| KARMA YOGA | ACTION |
| RAJA YOGA | CONSCIOUSNESS |

FIVE DIVISIONS OF YOGA

*Hatha yoga* helps the practitioner to gain fuller control over the functions of his physical body. In untrained man the conscious mind knows very little about what goes on below the level of consciousness. The conscious mind is like the tip of an iceberg, nine-tenths of which is submerged and out of reach. Our body is a mystery. We know practically nothing of what goes on down below and have no control over our own inner workings. All we know is that our moods change and our feelings of self change. We may feel happy or miserable for no reason we can discern. All these mood changes are due to processes taking place below the surface, but we have no control over these processes and thus are at the mercy of our inner chemistry. If something goes wrong with our liver, our whole outlook changes.

A student of hatha yoga gradually learns to understand what goes on below the surface. He learns consciously to perceive and control many processes that are ordinarily out of reach. He becomes the master of his body, instead of being its slave. This mastery over the body confers on the hatha yogi powers that seem extraordinary. Members of the Hillary expedition to the Himalayas were amazed to find a Nepalese pilgrim lightly clad and barefoot living in apparent comfort amidst the snows. They subjected the poor fellow to a whole battery of scientific tests, hoping to discover the secret of his extraordinary resistance to stress. Of course they discovered nothing. The secret was hatha yoga.

Western science, which is very backward in certain respects, has just recently discovered that rats can be trained to control certain autonomic functions and that even men, who in some ways are not as smart as rats, can be similarly trained. The scientists, of course, use whole batteries of electronic gadgets to provide what they call autonomic feedback. With these rather elaborate aids people can learn to control heart rate, stomach acidity, and other physical phenomena which hatha yogis have known how to control for centuries.

One of the chief benefits conferred by hatha yoga is a condition that might be described as superhealth. The hatha yogi is practically never ill. His functions are harmonized and he knows how to keep them harmonized. The regular practice of certain basic hatha yoga exercises is the finest recipe there is for perfect health. Unfortunately for modern man, who is very lazy and relies on some machine to make his efforts for him, the exercises are difficult to master and must be performed with unfailing regularity if they are to have any effect. This is true of all yoga exercises.

*Jnana yoga* is the yoga of the intellect. From the standpoint of jnana yoga, what man calls his mind is little more than an instrument for the creation of illusions. Before a person can even begin to approach reality he must learn to silence his ordinary mind, to stop the endless flow of associative thinking, the inner conversations, the schemings, dreamings, and babblings that keep him in a perpetual state of inner noise. In order really to think he must first learn to stop thoughts.

This exercise of stopping thoughts is so fundamental that it would be wrong to consider it only an aspect of jnana yoga. It is basic to all forms of yoga. What jnana yoga teaches is that man, besides having a lower mind that creates illusions, also has a higher mind. This higher mind is called in Sanskrit "buddhi." It is a faculty that man does not ordinarily use, which will enable him to penetrate the veil of maya created by the ordinary mind.

One of the things a student of jnana yoga learns first is a deep distrust for words and for verbal thinking. The lower mind, which is a horrendously inefficient piece of machinery, tends to become completely hypnotized by words. Some of the most disastrous conflicts in human history have resulted from this word hypnosis. Wars between the faithful and the infidels, the orthodox and the heretics, the communists and the fascists, were all squabbles about words. Time and again whole cultures have been ruined because of obscure theological arguments, defined in words that neither side could understand. The lower mind's tendency to word hypnosis, along with its extreme credulity and suggestibility, is one of the most disastrous defects of the human machine. Jnana yoga teaches man how to keep from getting entangled in words.

The student of jnana yoga, having learned to stop verbal thinking, next learns to use entirely different instruments for thought. These instruments take the form of certain pictures or diagrams. In Sanskrit the diagrams are called *yantra*. In transcendental magic they are called "arcana." The mandala shown earlier (Figure 4) is an example of such a diagram. There are many others. The Grand Arcanum of the tarot cards, for example, contains an enormous amount of information, though the cards are not complete in themselves. One of the quests of students of transcendental magic was to find the universal arcanum, the one supreme symbol that would give to the magician both power and knowledge. King Solomon's ring was supposed to have been inscribed with this great symbol, but the ring has been lost and the great symbol with it. In any case, jnana yoga teaches man to think in entirely new categories.

*Bhakti yoga* is the yoga of religious emotion. For certain people religious emotion is a very powerful force. Like most powerful forces, religious emotion can act either creatively or destructively. Some of the most disgusting manifestations of human cruelty have resulted from a combination of destructive religious emotion and the word hypnosis of the lower mind. The followers of three major religions—Christianity, Islam, and Judaism—have always been especially prone to this disease. Oceans of blood have been shed in the name of these religions. Christians slaughtered Moslems. Moslems slaughtered Christians, not to mention Hindus and Buddhists. Both slaughtered Jews, who would certainly have slaughtered back had they been better armed and organized.

All this destruction resulted from the fact that followers of these religions used different words for God and had different theories about his attributes, theories that none of them could prove and which were all equally erroneous. The function of bhakti yoga is to teach the practitioner to go beyond theories and to see God in all things. Above all, bhakti yoga trains man to transmute his negative emotions. The Sermon on the Mount is a treatise on bhakti yoga. It is a very difficult form of yoga. People do not want to give up their negative emotions. They want to indulge in them and justify them. And many aspects of our present-day culture encourage this indulgence by pouring out endless stories of violence and crime, which the young eagerly absorb even before they can talk.

*Karma yoga* is the yoga of action. It applies especially to the third stage of life, the stage of the householder. During this stage both men and women are necessarily involved in a lot of activity. As a result of this activity they tend to lose sight of their inner aims, to become totally preoccupied with externals, often very petty ones. Karma yoga teaches its practitioners how to remain detached in the midst of activity. It teaches that everything happens in accordance with certain laws, that men have very little control over events because they have very little understanding of these laws. The student is taught to regard himself as a vehicle through which certain forces operate. Unless he is on guard he has no control over these forces. They will compel him to do certain things even against his will. He begins to realize that he is a very small cog in a very big machine and that, if he wants to avoid being crushed, he must watch what he is doing. Yet karma yoga is based on a paradox. At the same time that it says, "Only he who is blinded by egoism thinks 'I' am the doer," it also demands that a person take responsibility for his actions, that he know what he is doing and why.

Finally there is *raja yoga*. The name implies that this is the king of the yogas. From some points of view it is. Raja yoga teaches that there are two aspects of man's being, the little personal self, or jiva, and the Great Self, or atman. In man's ordinary state of consciousness the petty personal self is all that man knows. He identifies with it completely. Its fears, hopes, likes, dislikes, and ambitions govern the course of his life. Raja yoga teaches that this bundle of personal prejudices is not the self at all. It teaches the student to see his life as a wave that comes into being, develops, reaches its peak, falls, sweeps up on the beach, returns to the ocean, and disappears. All waves return to the ocean from which they came. It would be absurd for a wave to think it had a separate identity. The ocean is vast and eternal, the waves are tiny and temporal. It is within man's power if he so chooses to transcend his petty personal consciousness and reblend with the greater whole from which these separate consciousnesses emerged. In so doing he returns intentionally to the source and takes part in an ascending movement of the cosmic process. But to do so a man must see that his ordinary consciousness, his ordinary sense of self, is illusory. He must see how he depends on the surrounding biosphere, how an exchange of energies makes his life possible. Eating, breathing, and receiving impressions begin to take on a new significance for him.

Raja yoga is especially suitable for people in the fourth stage of life. It prepares man to face his death. One who has fully mastered the techniques of raja yoga can leave his physical body at will. He does this by entering the state of samadhi, which is the equivalent of the first after-death state, the experiencing of the Clear Light of the Void. From this state he can either return to the physical body or simply shed it as a man sheds a worn-out garment.

I come now to the last subject of this talk, the drugs that affect the psyche, the so-called psychedelics. Can these drugs aid the process of psychotransformism? No general answer can be given to this question. It depends on which drug is used, how it is used, and by whom. Drug plants of the belladonna group, for instance, are traditionally the power plants of sorcerers. They give to the user the taste of power. Once he has had that taste, the user is apt to pursue power for its own sake. The crimson fly agaric appears to work in the same way, hence its popularity with Siberian shamans. These are all quite dangerous substances and are apt to destroy those who experiment with them carelessly.

Next there is the group of revelatory drugs, to which peyote, ayahuasca, cohoba, hashish, and LSD belong. They can, if taken under the right conditions, after careful preparation, reveal certain worlds that are normally hidden from man. Whether these worlds are perceived as beautiful or terrifying depends on set and setting. The drugs cannot possibly change a person's level of being, but they may change his perspective. He may, as a result of drug-induced revelations, become dissatisfied with ordinary life games. He may seek a guide and embark on the Way. Or he may merely become confused, lose the way altogether, and sink deeper and deeper into the

FIGURE 7

| DRUG | ORIGIN | ACTIVE PRINCIPLE |
|------|--------|------------------|
| DEVIL'S WEED | DATURA SPP. | SCOPOLAMINE |
| TOLOACHE | ATROPA BELLADONNA | ATROPINE |
| PEYOTE | LOPHOPHORA WILLIAMSII | MESCALINE |
| TEONANACATL | PSILOCYBE MEXICANA | PSILOCYBIN |
| AYAHUASCA | BANNISTERIOPSIS CAAPI | HARMALINE |
| EPENA | VIROLA CALOPHYLLOIDEA | DIMETHYLTRYPTAMINE (DMT) |
| COHOBA | PIPTADENIA PERIGRINA | DMT |
| SOMA | AMANITA MUSCARIA (?) | IBOTENIC ACID MUSCIMOL |
| KAVA | PIPER METHYSTICUM | KAWAIN DIHYDROMETHYSTICIN |
| NUTMEG | MYRISTICA FRAGRANS | ELEMICIN (?) |
| HASHISH | CANNABIS SATIVA | TETRAHYDROCANNABINOL |
| LSD | SYNTHETIC | D-LYSERGIC ACID DIETHYLAMIDE |
| DOM OR STP | SYNTHETIC | 4 METHYL-2, 5-DIMETHOXYAMPHETAMINE |

morass by taking drugs more and more often. It is these unfortunates who become slaves to drugs that have given the word *drug* its sinister connotations. We should bear in mind, however, that the drugs most commonly abused are not the revelatory drugs but those hoary old poisons alcohol and tobacco, which have led more people to a premature death than have all the revelatory drugs combined.

From the standpoint of psychotransformism the drugs are not of much value. Psychotransformism is a process demanding effort, like any other creative process. If a person wishes to master a difficult art, a difficult science, or a difficult physical feat such as swimming the English Channel or running the four-minute mile, he knows he must practice and train himself by constant effort. A concert pianist, for instance, may practice eight hours a day. One of the great concert pianists defined the importance of practice very clearly. "If I miss one day's practice I notice the difference. If I miss two days' practice my wife notices the difference. If I miss a week's practice even the audience notices the difference."

What would happen to such a master performer if he stopped practicing and began to take drugs because he thought that, in some miraculous way, they would improve his technique? Obviously his power would disappear. He would lose his mastery over the instrument and drift off into a world of illusions. Exactly the same thing happens to any follower of the Way who imagines he can take a shortcut by using drugs. He merely lands himself in a world of illusions. He may think he is getting results, but the results are imaginary. He is in fact moving backward, sinking into a morass from which it will become more and more difficult to escape. In the end he will sink so deeply that he will not be able to escape at all.

# Robert S. de Ropp: *Questions*

*Question:* Could you comment on the theory that the pineal gland contains enzymes that produce serotonin-like psychedelic substances, and that they do so under natural conditions in some animals, and maybe even in man? It seems to me to have an interesting connection with the idea of enlightenment, because the pineal seems to be in some way connected with perception of light and dark cycles and controlling the animal's biorhythms between the light and dark cycles. It could be that some of the metaphors of enlightenment come from the idea that under certain conditions the pineal is stimulated to produce these substances which create, in some way, the sensation of light from an extraordinary source.

*Dr. de Ropp:* There's been a great deal of nonsense written about that little entity called the pineal gland. Is there another question?

*Question:* Could you speak about what we are practicing in the development of consciousness?

*Answer:* Now *there's* a good question!

Practice, practice. You see, if you want to have the whole thing down pat, I'll give you four principles which will enable you to attain the heights—the highest heights. Listen carefully. The first one: stop thoughts and be here now. Got that one? The second one: learn to transform your poisons into honey. This refers to the transmutation of negative emotions—the most difficult part of the work. Got that? Now the third one: substitute intentional doing for accidental happening. Fantastically difficult! Even if I raise my hand, it can be intentional or it can just raise itself. And finally, the most difficult one of all: do nothing unnecessary. Whenever I say this to members of my group they say, "Oh, but how am I to know whether it's unnecessary or not?" It can also be formulated: avoid unnecessary karma. We entangle ourselves unnecessarily in all sorts of useless activities, particularly the so-called "social life," which drains us of our energies, exalts our false egos, and generally damages us. So the fourth principle helps us to avoid getting tied up in that kind of thing. That's the best thing I've said yet. If you just remember that, that's all you need to know.

*Question:* What happens when you get enlightened?

*Answer:* Well, the Buddha said when he got enlightened, "Really and truly, it's not worthwhile bothering to try to enlighten anybody else—this bunch of idiots would never understand it in the first place, and I'd much prefer just to sit here and enjoy my enlightenment." Then some god came down and said, "Look, wouldn't you like to change your mind?" There was a certain amount of discussion that went on and finally the Buddha said, "Well, maybe there are a few people around who are not completely stupid, so I'll go out and see if I can find them." And that's what he did after he was enlightened—went around teaching others. But you don't have to do that.

*Question:* I wonder why he did it?

*Answer:* He probably regretted it.

*Question:* How do you go about finding a teacher?

*Answer:* Well, you can look in the Yellow Pages. . . . How *do* you? I mean, how did I? I'll tell you. I was first of all interested in theosophy, and then I started reading about those mahatma letters that came through the ceiling, you know? And I was a scientist. "After all, that sort of thing can't go on—it can't happen." Then I met Ouspensky. And there was something about Ouspensky I immediately liked. He was always, *always* saying, "Believe nothing I say. Don't accept anything. This teaching, this Fourth Way teaching, is based on understanding, not on faith." Those matches struck on my box. Understanding—yes. "If you don't understand it, do nothing. But wait—try to understand." Now this tradition is still being carried on, and if you can find that kind of teacher, he can help you. But this only appeals to skeptics like myself. The starry-eyed believer will follow anybody. I honestly believe we could train a dog, and have him presented as the Perfect Master, and I honestly believe he'd get a following!

*Question:* Will you explain more about changing poisons into honey?

*Answer:* "Love your enemies"—this whole Christian teaching —"resist not evil," "turn the other cheek," is based on that principle. It is fantastically difficult because everything in our culture tells us to do the exact opposite: "Don't transform your poisons into honey, but transform them into more poison— worse poison. Justify your negative emotions. Revel in them. And if you can't find any negative emotions of your own, just watch TV."

What are you going to do? It's terribly difficult. . . . No, seriously, the first step in this transmutation is to realize that these negative emotions are not justified, and they're neither pleasurable nor profitable, and they don't do you any good. You have to talk to your emotional center with your intellectual center. Your emotional center is very fast and rather stupid. Your intellectual center is slow, but more intelligent. So your intellectual center says, "Hey, hold it now. Wait a minute here. What's all this going on? It's not necessary—it's not useful." Little by little you really come to see that it's not necessary and not useful and then you gradually begin to transmute, actually change. It's a truly great moment.

*Question:* Do you feel that your training as a scientist and, in general, all the biochemical study of the brain has much importance in understanding the "Way" that you described and talked about? Would you regard it as necessary?

*Answer: No!* I wouldn't want everybody to train in neurochemistry. That would be asking too much. But what you have to understand is this: events at a molecular level can tremendously influence your entire feeling of self. You may wake up one morning feeling perfectly awful. The real reason is that there's something slightly amiss in your chemistry. So, we are a hierarchy of cosmoses, if you like. Starting way down at the subatomic level and going up through the atoms, the molecules, the cells, the organs, and, finally, the totality. And each level influences the level above.

I remember when LSD appeared on the scene. I couldn't believe it! How could any drug be so effective at the level of one hundred fifty *micro*grams? Fantastically small dose. So of course I had to try the stuff. And lo and behold! Strange events and strange feelings started to happen, and I thought, "Good grief! What's going on in that brain?" It showed me in a very, very clear way how this tiny trace of a chemical—a *minute* amount—was completely altering my whole sense of self. So there are events at a molecular level that totally change your sense of self.

*Question:* How do you see the molecular description of the further stages—or at least one or two of the stages that you described as on the Way—such as objective man? Do you feel that if you looked in the brain and analyzed it chemically, you would be able to . . .

*Answer:* No sir!! The chemist—the biochemist—can only go a very little way. In *Drugs and the Mind* ° I've compared him to

° Grove Press, New York, 1960.

a burglar trying to crack a very large safe with a toothpick. He's very poorly armed, and he can't go very far. In order to go beyond the stage of biochemistry you have to start using alchemy. Alchemy is the method whereby you use your own sensations and your own awarenesses and your own feelings to study the transmutation of substances in your own being. Neoalchemy is the basis of Gurdjieff's teachings.

*Question:* There's a school of thought represented by people such as Alan Watts and Krishnamurti who say that the whole business of a path or applied effort to attain enlightenment is in some sense illusory, just a sophisticated ego game. I wonder: is it not one's ego that is making the effort to attain something?

*Answer:* Yes, I suppose it is, but there's a very odd thing about this particular kind of effort. It's sort of effortless. If you sit around like Rodin's Thinker, all hunched up, you get nowhere. You have to let it flow. First of all, the idea that *I* am going to attain anything—the moment that occurs, that's the end. *I* am not going to attain anything. *I* am going to disappear. But something else is going to appear in "my" place, and this is part of the atman, part of the Greater Self. If you go about it in this way, I think you'll avoid falling into the trap that I once called the Personal Salvation Syndrome. If you're hooked on personal salvation, you've had it.

*Question:* In the light of what you said about how chemistry affects the sense of self: when do you seek a doctor, when do you seek a psychiatrist, and when do you seek a teacher?

*Answer:* "When do you seek a psychiatrist?" I never seek psychiatrists. I've seen too much of them. They either give you pills or they lay you out on a couch and ask you to tell them all about your childhood sweetheart. I think when you're really in a very bad way—when you are psychologically upset and your functioning is very bad—you're going to go to a doctor. But if you're perfectly healthy and normal and you've got the idea that there is something beyond this, beyond your ordinary experiences, you'll probably go around looking for a teacher, wouldn't you?

*Question:* You seem to believe that man is in a rather bad way. He has this brain which Nature has given him, which is of very little use. Yet this brain must still somehow suit Nature's purpose. Perhaps all of mankind could change, or be changed?

*Answer:* It would be very nice if it happened. But since the beginning of time we come across these statements that very few find the Path—out of a hundred thousand, one or two will find the Way. I can only tell you what Ouspensky used to tell us—that man lives under the law of seeds. Take, for instance, an oak tree. It probably produces millions of acorns during the course of its long existence. How many of those acorns are going to grow into an oak? Nature, in the case of man, has produced an enormous amount of human material—human biomatter, which gets bigger all the time, growing like a cancer. Out of it, a minute proportion develops. Tiny, minute. Tiny fraction of one percent. You say, "Why on earth should Nature go to the trouble of creating this huge mass of stuff just to get this tiny little quantity of higher matter?" That's the way Nature works.

*Question:* Your opening remarks seemed to indicate that a tiny amount of chemical was all that was needed—

*Answer:* Nature just needs a tiny amount of this higher man—she doesn't need a lot.

*Question:* Are you familiar with Kundalini yoga? Apparently there's energy derived from the base of the spine, which travels up through the back of the spinal chord and stimulates the brain. Do you feel there is some biochemical foundation for that—for Kundalini?

*Answer:* Well, the whole theory of the chakras and these energy substances is very, very far beyond the reach of biochemistry. The biochemist is handicapped, since, apart from everything else, he can't experiment with human beings. He has to work with rats.

*Question:* There's cerebrospinal fluid—

*Answer:* The cerebrospinal fluid is just a cushion, that's all.

*Question:* But it does seem to have some sort of flow, or—I mean it's connected . . .

*Answer:* It circulates, but that doesn't mean a thing. You can't equate the chakras with the cerebrospinal fluid. They are certain centers of energy that aren't in the ordinary body at all.

*Question:* But couldn't possibly some small, minute quantities of a chemical be secreted into the cerebrospinal fluid at some location—or not at any particular location—and have an effect throughout the brain?

*Answer:* Yes, of course they could. But I'm telling you that the biochemist wouldn't be able to detect them. He cannot possibly pick up these things.

*Question:* But couldn't one experiment by putting chemicals into the system and detecting the effect?

*Answer:* Well, yes, if you can find anybody fool enough to submit to such experiments. But the yogi who's practicing these things *knows* from his direct experience that something is happening. He doesn't need to be a biochemist.

# Drugs, Yoga, and Psychotransformism

*Question:* Could you comment on the theory that serotonin is a common element in schizophrenia and yogic experiences?

*Answer:* All this is largely hogwash. Damn biochemistry! Serotonin occurs in the brain; it occurs in a lot of things. Serotonin—so much has been attributed to serotonin. Anything the biochemist doesn't understand, he'll say, "Oh yes, that's because there's too much serotonin." And somebody will turn around and say, "On the contrary, it's because there's too little serotonin."

*Question:* You don't think it's common to all these experiences; you don't think it's the common element in schizophrenia and yogic experiences?

*Answer:* No, no, no. Schizophrenia is the result of a poison, which is brewed by the incorrect metabolism of dopa. But I'm not going into that—that's biochemistry.

*Question:* You mentioned Koestler's description of the modern brain and ancient brain in man. It's as though man has two TV sets in him which are not hooked up together. What happens to this seeker if he travels the path and climbs the mountain? Does he straighten out his two sets?

*Answer:* He gets the crocodile on speaking terms with the horse, and the horse and the crocodile on speaking terms with the man, and he knows who's who in the zoo.

*Question:* What is the significance of the Fourth Way?

*Answer:* Ouspensky used to give six preliminary lectures on that, which I think have been published in a book.* I never read them, but I heard the lectures. More than once.

* *The Psychology of Man's Possible Evolution,* Alfred A. Knopf, New York, 1954.

*Question:* Why do you feel that this kind of work is best approached or best attempted in a rural atmosphere, rather than metropolitan?

*Answer:* That simply happens to be a preference of mine. But you know, you are dependent upon the country. You have to get your food from the biosphere—it doesn't all grow in the A&P supermarkets. It's growing in the dirt. And we are dirt. And the dirt under our feet will one day cover our graves. I like to get my thing together. I grow my own vegetables and I live off what I grow in my own garden. And what I can't get from the garden, I get from the ocean. And that way of life appeals to me. It doesn't necessarily appeal to everybody.

*Question:* You talked about the proper ways of prayer. How would you find that and what are some methodologies?

*Answer:* Well, there are two kinds of prayer. There's the "gimme" type, which addresses the higher powers as if they were a sort of supermarket and says, "Well, look, I need some of this and I need some of that and I could do with a little of this and please let me off the hook with my income-tax troubles and that's why I've come to pray." Then there's another kind of prayer which involves centering and getting into touch with this inner temple. You can't describe it, because it's beyond words. It's just something you have to experience. "Stop thoughts. Be here now." That's the beginning, the first principle.

*Question:* How do you stop thoughts?

*Answer:* How do you stop thoughts? "Stop." They start again. "Stop." And they start again. You have a watchman at the door so the people who come in and out can be controlled, you see? You probably know Gurdjieff's comparison between a sleeping man and a conveyance. There's a horse, a coachman, a carriage, and someone in the carriage. In sleeping man—in the ordinary "waking" state of consciousness, so-called—the horse goes anywhere it wants, the coachman is drunk or asleep, the carriage is in rotten repair, and anybody can get into the carriage and drive anywhere! That's our ordinary state. Any "I"—and we have many "I's"—can get up and say *I'm* going to do this, and does it. And the other "I's" maybe have to pay for that stupidity for the rest of their lives. The person who should be traveling in the carriage is the master, but the master won't even get into that carriage until: first, the carriage has been fixed; second, the horse has been disciplined; and third, the coachman wakes up and begins to take orders from the master. All this involves a lot of work. And this stopping thoughts is part of this work.

*Question:* How do you see contemporary science as it's now developing, especially in terms of some of the things that are beginning to come out about holistic theory and hierarchy? Do you see that as something that can *aid* in what you're calling transformism, or do you see that as an impediment in terms of the secularization of sacred ideas?

*Answer:* Oh, all this stuff is words—it's just professorial chitchat. People write books about it; it doesn't mean a thing.

*Question:* You've obviously read very widely in this field and you've had a great deal of personal experience in the areas you've talked about. I'm wondering what the distillation of your experience has been: what do you regard as very personally yours in this whole area?

*Answer:* Nothing personal at all. I haven't got any personal feelings about this thing. It's very old, and it's very well known, and it's been around a long time.

*Question:* If men are likened to acorns, what determines, for any one man, whether he can develop into a tree?

*Answer:* It depends where the acorn alights and whether the acorn's alive to begin with. There are dead acorns and living acorns. Not every acorn will germinate. But you can see when you look at an oak that the acorn that drops and stays right under it doesn't have much of a chance. But if a squirrel takes that acorn and doesn't eat it but buries it in some nice little spot where there aren't any oaks, it can grow. So find the right spot!

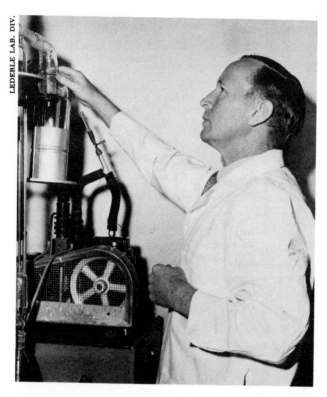

*Robert S. de Ropp*, Ph.D., is a noted biochemist whose primary research has been done in the field of brain chemistry and drugs that affect human behavior. Among his best-known books are *Drugs and the Mind*, *The Master Game*, and *Church of the Earth*.

# MAN'S SEARCH
# FOR
# ULTIMATE MEANING

## Viktor E. Frankl

To understand the relationship between psychiatry and religion in the world today, it is necessary to realize that, in essence, they move on different levels and aim at quite different results. The goal of psychiatry is mental health, but the goal of religion is something entirely apart from mental health. Whatever else you may call it, *re-ligio* literally means the re-establishing of the link between man and deity. The word for this in the West is *salvation*.

Mental health and salvation: two quite different goals, and two quite different processes that lead to these goals. But as to the by-products, the unintentional side effects of these processes, something quite interesting happens. Religion, without striving for it, doubtlessly contributes much to mental health by offering a man security and the feeling of being anchored in the Absolute. And, strangely, something comparable happens in any effective process of psychotherapy. For, although the psychiatrist as such does not, and must not, attempt to affect the religious life of his patient, one of the by-products of a good psychotherapeutic treatment is the re-establishment in man of a link to deity.

In my book *Psychotherapy and Existentialism*° I described

° Simon and Schuster, New York, 1968.

at length the case of a painter who came to me because of her difficulties in working as an artist. Without my intending it, without my even being aware of it, after several weeks she became capable not only of working, but also of praying and of engaging in religious meditation. Whatever personal views that I or any psychiatrist may have about religion or religious experience, it is important for us to see to it that our particular psychiatric approach, in my case logotherapy, remains *applicable* to every patient, the atheist as well as the believer. I also feel obliged to see to it that my methodology remains *useable* in the hands of every psychiatrist or psychologist, regardless of whether or not he has a religious orientation.

But even more important, one also has to see to it that the door to transcendence and *religious self-actualization*, the passageway out of the secular realm within which we move when we are striving for mental health, be left open and not be narrowed or blocked by the therapy or the therapist.

It was more than fifty years ago, in 1924, that my first psychiatric paper was published in the *International Journal of Psychoanalysis* upon the explicit invitation of Sigmund Freud. And so I bear witness for what was going on then: the way in which psychoanalysts and psychotherapists dismissed the religious life of a patient as a mere personal "hangup," and, more generally, how they explained away *all* religion as being, in Freud's words, the "obsessive-compulsive collective neurosis of mankind." "God," said Freud, "is nothing but the projection of an individual's father image." Perhaps this sort of approach to religion is no longer in favor among psychiatrists —I hope not. But any such restricted and rigid psychodynamic interpretation of the phenomenon of religion is liable merely to explain it away by forcing it onto the Procrustean bed of scientific reductionism.

A real interpretation of religion is possible, but it requires a methodology, a mode of analysis, that is not psychodynamic but phenomenological. Such an analysis must be unbiased and unprejudiced by the sort of preconceived patterns of interpretation that are the stock in trade on most American campuses and on the American analytical couch—and here I am speaking both of the behaviorist approaches and the numerous psychodynamic approaches. The core of the phenomenological method is the demand to perceive human phenomena at their face value, a demand that requires extraordinary intellectual integrity and persistent sensitivity of feeling. This is *empiricism in the noblest sense of the word*, not in the sense restricted to so-called empirical, scientific methods. Because it is experiential—that is, because it depends solely on our own experience and does not try to deny any part of this experience by pressing it onto a bed of Procrustes—it adheres to what Henri Bergson once called *"les données immédiates de la conscience,"* the immediate data of our own consciousness. Of course, we need to be careful not to confuse this approach with the smuggling in of a preconceived private *Weltanschauung* and philosophy of life, which is often sold under the guise of down-to-earth, strictly empirical research.

The phenomenon of religion is of special interest to logotherapy; indeed, the very word *logos* signifies "meaning." The whole discipline of logotherapy pivots around man's search for meaning or, as we are accustomed to saying, man's will to meaning.

I cannot discuss here all the research that has been done and all the evidence that has been accumulated showing that the will to meaning is a real, primordial motivating force in human nature. What I do want to point out—and this is something many people feel—is that this will to meaning is increasingly frustrated in the conditions of modern life. So much is this so that during the last decade this "existential frustration" has taken over the place that sexual frustration occupied during the time of Freud. Similarly as regards patients suffering from the effects of inferiority feelings: we encounter far fewer than existed during the days of Alfred Adler. Instead, we find in our patients an abysmal feeling of futility, meaninglessness, and emptiness, which I have termed the "existential vacuum."

Man, unlike animals, is not totally informed by drives and instincts as to what he *must* do. But modern man is unique in that, unlike people in former times, he lacks the traditions that tell him what he *should* do. And so now he is at a loss. Knowing neither what he *must* do nor what he *should* do, it often seems that he no longer even knows what he really *wants* to do. And the result is either that he just wishes to do what other people are doing, conformism, or else he simply does what other people tell him to do, totalitarianism. This existential vacuum forms the mass neurosis, the ill, the ailment of our time.

In a letter to Princess Bonaparte, Freud once wrote that "at the moment a man questions the meaning and value of his life he is sick." I cannot subscribe to this view. And as a case in point I would cite the example of a professor at the University of Vienna who was· referred to me by the department of cardiology because of his depressions. This man also doubted the meaning of his life. He was, in fact, suffering from endogenous depressions—that is to say, depressions that are primarily organic in origin. But the experience of doubting the meaning of his life occurred only during the intervals when he was emotionally normal. Thus there can even exist a mutually exclusive relationship between disease, emotional disease, and despair, existential despair.

Now, to respond to the question: "How can a doctor, a psychiatrist, a physician, or a counselor in any of the helping professions give meaning to a client, a patient?" We cannot give meaning to anyone. Meaning can only be found, discovered; it cannot be invented. And it must be discovered by oneself, by one's own conscience—because conscience is the only instrument we have that can discover meaning in life, a discovery that operates in a manner analogous to gestalt perceptions. Kurt Lewin once said that in each situation of life there is a gestalt, a requirement, a factor of demand. Max Wertheimer also spoke of the requirements of a given situation in terms of a demand quality. He added, however, that this quality of demand is objective in nature—that is, it is always already there and needs only to be found, perceived, not created.

These are gestalt psychologists speaking. A gestalt is perceived as a figure against a background; but a meaning gestalt, I would say, is perceived as a *possibility* against the background of *reality*. I immediately perceive, here and now, in a given situation, confronted with this particular reality, that there is a possibility for me, there is something I can and must do. This is the meaning inherent and dormant in the given situation. And the business of finding it, of scenting it out, so to speak, is the task allotted to conscience.

These possibilities are always unique and unprecedented. Thus, it is only in a given situation, at the actual moment, that a person—who is also unique—can do something in or about this situation, can fulfill the unique possibility and meaning of the moment. From this it follows that even though the sacred traditions of the West are on the wane and even though the values held dear by our society throughout history are disappearing, meanings are always possible as long as conscience exists. Whereas values are transmitted through traditions because they are shared by peoples and generations, meanings are always unique and always appear in a unique situation calling out, as it were, to a unique human individual. They cannot be transmitted, not even by a sacred tradition. They have always, again and again, to be discovered by our personal, lonely conscience.

So it doesn't make sense to ask anyone, "What is the meaning of our life?" It's like asking Bobby Fischer, "What is the best move in chess?" He would answer, "It depends on the given constellation of the game and the specific skills of the particular players." It is this uniqueness that accounts for the load of responsible-ness laid on our shoulders throughout life. And there is nothing that can be found in the whole literature of mankind that can match what Hillel said two thousand years ago. You may find it in the *Pirke Abot*, the

*Wisdom of the Fathers*: "If not I for myself, who then? And being for myself, what am I? And if not now, when?"

"If not I for myself, who then?" The uniqueness of my person is involved. "And if not now, when?" The uniqueness of the situation is involved. Everything, every situation, every possibility in life is transitory. But once we have transformed a possibility into a reality, have actualized it, have fulfilled its potential meaning, we have rescued it into the past where nothing and nobody can ever deprive us of it. It has been saved from transitoriness by being safely deposited in the storehouse of the past.

"Being for myself, what am I?" This refers to perhaps the most fundamental characteristic of human existence, which I have termed "self-transcendence." Human reality, by virtue of its self-transcendent quality, always points to, is directed to, is related to, something that is not itself, something or someone other than itself: either a meaning to fulfill—out there, in the world—or another human being lovingly to encounter. Self-transcendence is lived out by serving a cause or loving a person. And to the very extent to which we love other persons or serve causes other than ourselves, we actualize ourselves by way of a side effect. *We become more human and more ourselves by forgetting ourselves and giving ourselves.*

Our eyes are self-transcendent. The power of my eye to perceive the surrounding world is inextricably dependent on its incapacity to see itself. And should I actually see anything of my own eye—for instance, a halo around a light—it is my glaucoma or cataract that I see. Only the diseased eye perceives something of itself. The normally functioning eye perceives the world precisely, because it cannot see anything of itself. And that is self-transcendence. To the extent that a man is preoccupied with anything within himself—pleasure, prestige, happiness, and so forth—to that extent he is no longer really functioning and existing on a human level. Humanness is contingent on his forgetting and overlooking himself, as the eye overlooks and forgets itself. "Being for myself, what am I?" I am not really living out my humanness.

We have been speaking of the uniqueness of meanings. From this it follows that the meaning of life—the meaning in any life situation—is constantly changing. But it is *never missing; life never lacks meaning,* though it is up to me to discover it. And there are three main avenues to this discovery. First, by doing a deed or creating a work. Second, by experiencing something or someone beyond oneself, experiencing another person in his very uniqueness through loving. As for the third avenue to meaning, we can best understand it by realizing that even if a man has to face an implacable fate—for instance, an incurable disease—there is still meaning available, literally up to his last breath, to life's last moment. Because then a man may bear witness to the specifically human potential at its best, which is to turn tragedy into triumph, to transform one's predicament into an achievement on the human level. In other words, due to the very uniqueness, the ever-changing but never-missing quality of meaning, life's meaningfulness is unconditional. Life remains meaningful under any conditions and circumstances.

A review in the *American Journal of Psychiatry* once praised logotherapy for its "unconditional belief in the unconditional meaningfulness of life." But is this triad of values—creation, experience, and transformation—really just a belief?

I was a young student when I first grasped this trichotomy— the three avenues leading to unconditional meaning—and I confess I did so on a purely intuitive basis. But during the last five or six years ample evidence has been offered by dozens of dissertations, by strictly empirical research, and by statistics covering thousands of subjects, all showing that people do find meaning in these three ways and that, in the final analysis, there is always a meaning available, literally up to the last moment. These studies also show that such meaning is available to people irrespective of age, sex, I.Q., educational background, outer circumstances, and inner character makeup and, interestingly enough, irrespective of whether one is religious or not and, if one is religious, whether one belongs to this or that denomination.

And so now we come specially to the subject of religion, which we may define not simply as man's search for meaning but rather as his search for ultimate meaning. Now, the more comprehensive a meaning is, the less comprehensible it turns out to be. And as for ultimate meaning, it is completely beyond comprehension, at least on merely intellectual or scientific grounds. What is required is an emotional approach in the noblest sense, involving not merely what goes under the name of "affect," but an approach that reaches down to the existential foundations of our human reality where we can answer to life from the depth and wholeness of our being and not just from one aspect of our personalities, where we identify ourselves as scientists, for example, or psychiatrists, or partners in love.

Because ultimate meaning is located in a different, a higher, dimension, it is accessible to finite being only through the mediation of symbol. Let us consider this idea of the "higher dimension." Certainly, no moral judgment is implied by the phrase *a higher dimension is simply a more inclusive dimension*. If, for example, you take a two-dimensional square and extend it vertically so that it becomes a three-dimensional cube, then you may say that the square is included in the cube. Anything occurring in the square on the two-dimensional level will be contained as well in the cube. And nothing that takes place in the square can contradict what occurs in the higher dimension of the cube. The higher dimension does not exclude; it includes. In the same way, a secular, scientifically established truth can never contradict a genuine religious truth, because real religion moves in a higher dimension. Religious truth includes scientific truth. Between the various levels of truth there can be no mutual exclusiveness, no real contradiction, for the higher includes the lower.

Let me try to make this more understandable by turning to some ideas from the book *Chance and Necessity*° by the molecular biologist and Nobel laureate Jacques Monod. In this

° Alfred A. Knopf, New York, 1971.

FIGURE 1

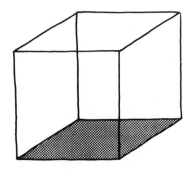

book Monod argues that all life results from the interaction of chance mutations and the forces of natural selection. For him, the idea of pure chance lies at the root of all evolution. This idea is, in his own words, "the only one conceivable because it is the only one compatible with the facts of observation and experience, and nothing permits us to suppose that our conceptions on this point will have to or even be able to be revised."

Now what is Monod doing? He strictly forbids us to entertain the possibility of a dimension other than that of molecular biology. He believes that only molecular biology can explain life, and that beyond the dimension of molecular biology nothing does or can exist. Such is the *a priori* philosophy of M. Monod. And it has nothing whatever to do with his or anyone else's findings in the field of molecular biology. Is it because he has been awarded the Nobel Prize that he believes that whatever ideas he offers under the name of science are not only true but exclusively and absolutely true? In any case, it is not worthy of a scientist to deny *a priori* the possibility of another dimension, especially if this denial is based on a private or personal philosophy.

The true scientist may not deny *a priori* the possibility of another dimension, nor should the religionist deny the reality that is scientifically established. There is no mutual exclusiveness between different dimensions, one of which includes the other. For discoveries made in one dimension of reality are simply encompassed by the truths of the higher dimension. And this holds for the sciences of the psyche as well, whether it be the findings of a Skinner or a Freud. At a certain level, their findings are sound and correct, but only at a certain level.

Thus, our problem is not that so many scientists are specializing but that so many specialists are generalizing!

We may say that a specialist such as M. Monod is moving in a particular plane. As a molecular biologist, he sees mutations, random events with no meaning behind or above them. For him, these mutations are disconnected; there is no meaningful pattern to relate them. But it may well be that what appears on the scientific level of biology as disconnected single points without any meaning beyond themselves is simply the result of the orthogonal interaction of two different dimensions, the horizontal plane of science being cut through by the vertical plane of a higher dimension. In the illustration below, for

FIGURE 2

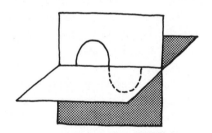

example, a sine curve in one dimension might very well intersect the horizontal plane in a seemingly meaningless pattern. Similarly, there could very well be a higher or deeper meaning behind the "chance" mutations described by the molecular biologist. Certainly, we cannot deny such a possibility *a priori*.

I have privately argued for hours at a time with Konrad Lorenz about this possibility, and he agrees that it is conceivable. Of course, as a neo-Darwinian operating within the plane of biology, he is simply not aware of anything in nature pointing to teleology, or inherent purpose. For him there is no meaning, no goal, no direction behind the movement of life. However, because he is not a reductionist, he does not *a priori* exclude the possibility that teleology might exist in another dimension. Thus, our scientists need to have more than good theories. They need to be wise as well. And wisdom I define in the following way: "knowledge plus the awareness of its limitations."

We who practice logotherapy also have to be aware of its limitations. I do not claim that it is a panacea. But it does help us look at the problems of life from another dimension, a more inclusive, "higher" dimension.

I remember when I was on my first lecture tour around the world in 1957. The American audiences would say, "Dr. Frankl, you are offering something quite novel and unprecedented." But when I went to Asia they told me exactly the contrary: "After all, Dr. Frankl, what you are offering us is very old. It's nothing but a modern version of the eternal and perennial wisdom contained in our ancient traditions." And I suppose they are right. In my own books I do sometimes make reference to Lao-tse, the Upanishads, or the Vedanta, for example. And I have published a paper in which I discuss a case handled by a Zen Buddhist psychiatrist in order to show the many parallels between logotherapy and Zen. At the same time, many studies have been made pointing out the similarities between logotherapy and Morita therapy, the famous Japanese method in which Zen Buddhism plays a decisive role. Even Shinto priests and Zen masters themselves have pointed out the parallels between my approach and theirs. This I cannot really judge, since I am no expert in this area.

But the most rewarding experience in this respect occurred two years ago at United States International University, when three Zen Buddhist monks in their yellow robes attended my lectures. At one point I called them over and asked them,

"Why do you attend my lectures? I cannot imagine that I have anything to offer you which is not already contained in your ancient scriptures."

They patiently let me finish speaking and then one of them said, "Dr. Frankl, in your classes we learn Zen Buddhism."

But as Johannes Schultz, the founder of the autogenic training methodology, once said, "There are no Christian, Moslem, Jewish, or Buddhist neuroses and psychoses; and therefore there cannot be such a thing as Buddhist or Christian or any other form of religious psychotherapy."

Then how are you Americans going to respond to all these psychological methods and teachings now pouring in upon you from the Orient? That, after all, is the main question you are asking. And I think there is an opportunity in this situation, but also a great danger.

For example, when people ask me about the main differences between European and American culture, I usually point out that while Americans try to pick up the best from Europe and transplant it onto their own soil, we Europeans on the contrary take the worst from America and simply proceed to ape it. Now, why shouldn't it be possible for Americans also to select the best, the perennial wisdom, from the Asian religions? Why shouldn't you borrow techniques and concepts that can truly help you? It would be foolish if you did otherwise. Yet I would like to voice a note of caution and skepticism.

I am against the blind transplanting of religious concepts, mainly because, as I see it, Western religion is a profoundly personal religion. And I believe that it will become ever more personalized, until finally every individual arrives at his own personal mode, his own personal language, when addressing himself to deity. And this even holds, in a way, for Asian religions. The following passage is from the wonderfully pointed book by Gordon Allport *The Individual and His Religion*. He is speaking of the "varying conceptions of deity held by different individuals and by one and the same individual at different periods of time." This statement mirrors what we have been speaking of as the uniqueness of meaning.

> When we need affection [says Allport], God is love; knowledge, He is omniscient; consolation, He granteth peace that passeth understanding. When we have sinned, He is the Redeemer; when we need guidance, the Holy Spirit. Divine attributes plainly conform to the panorama of desire, although the individual is seldom aware that his approach to his deity is determined by his present needs.
> An interesting rite in the Hindu tradition here comes to mind. Around the age of sixteen or eighteen, the Hindu youth receives from his teacher a name for God which all his life long shall serve this youth as a private instrument for prayer and for binding himself to the deity. In this custom, Hinduism recognizes that the temperament, needs and capacities of the initiate himself must in large part determine his approach to religious verities. . . . In this practice we have a rare instance of an institutional religion recognizing the ultimate individuality of the religious sentiment. . . .
> In India it is not enough that each individual should have a name for the deity suited to his own personal needs; it is also strictly advised that this name be kept secret even from one's bosom friend and from one's spouse. In the last analysis each person confronts his deity in solitude, and it is thought well to symbolize this fact, especially in over-crowded households and communities, with the seal of secrecy.*

Now, this personalization of religion is so much of a need that I question whether one can speak *of* God at all. I believe that one can really only speak *to* God. Wittgenstein once said, "Whereof one cannot speak, thereof one must be silent." I would translate this statement from agnostic into theistic

* Gordon Allport, *The Individual and His Religion* (New York: The Macmillan Co., 1952), pp. 10–11.

terminology by saying, "To Him of Whom one cannot speak, to Him one must pray." Prayer is always personal. *Prayer*, the addressing of oneself to deity, is never a station-to-station but always a *person-to-person* call. It's more expensive.

This person-to-person relationship was sharply envisaged, of course, by Martin Buber in his concept of the "I-Thou" relationship and in his belief that the fundamental agenda of the human spirit is carried out by way of dialogue. Let me, therefore, offer you a definition of God that I arrived at when I was fifteen years old; I offer it as a strictly operational definition.

I can visualize the precise street corner in Vienna where this came to me on my way home from school. I said to myself, "In the final analysis, *God is the partner of our most intimate soliloquies.* What may seem to be only a monologue is actually a dialogue with God." As I would put it now: God is He Who is the partner of your monologues whenever you speak to yourself in ultimate solitude and sincerity, without being distracted by any, so to say, earthly interests. If you are really sincere and speak to yourself, then the Being Whom you are actually addressing may justifiably be called God. This is an operational definition inasmuch as it is this side of the dichotomy in which the atheist and agnostic diverge from the believer.

But do any atheists really exist? This is questionable. In my book *The Unconscious God*,\* I offer some empirical, clinical evidence to show that even so-called atheists have strong, although unconscious, religious feelings. And these feelings are so deeply imbedded that even in cases of psychopathology there is evidence for their existence. I quote from the report by a patient of mine who was suffering from severe endogenous depression.

> In the mental hospital, I was locked in a cage like an animal. No one came when I called, begging to be taken to

\* Simon and Schuster, New York, 1975.

the bathroom, and I finally had to succumb to the inevitable. Blessedly, I was given daily shock treatment, insulin shock and was sufficiently drugged so that I lost most of the next several weeks. [It is absolutely justifiable to administer electroshock therapy and drugs in cases of endogenous depression because *these* depressions really originate in the realm of biochemistry.] But in the darkness I had acquired a sense of my own unique mission in the world. I knew then, as I know now, that I must have been spared for some reason, however small. . . . It's something that only I can do and it is vitally important that I do it. And because in the darkest moment of my life, when I lay abandoned as an animal in a cage, when because of the forgetfulness induced by electro-shock treatment, I could not call out to Him—yet, He was there. In the solitary darkness of the pit, where man had abandoned me, He was there. When I did not know His name, He was there. God was there.

So concludes this note from her diary.

Now, why did I speak of my skepticism and urge caution about transplanting Asian religious teachings to Western countries? It has to do with a particular trait common to Americans and very noticeable to Europeans traveling through this country. As soon as we arrive here, people command us to "just relax, enjoy yourself, be happy." Everywhere we go we are confronted with the manipulative approach to human phenomena. "Be happy, just relax." Of course, this is impossible. The more you try to relax, the more tense you become. Here, for example, is an excerpt from a research report by a student of mine in California. He was conducting experiments in electromyography by means of a technique that enables one to read the exact degree of muscle tension of the subject:

The electro-myograph was recording at a constantly high level (50 micro-amperes) until I told the subject, Steve, that he would probably never learn to relax and should resign himself to the fact that he would always be tense—"a lousy relaxer," as it were. A few minutes later, Steve stated, "Oh hell, I give up"—at which point the meter immediately dropped to a low level (10 micro-amperes from a level of 50) with such speed that I thought the unit had become disconnected. For the following sessions Steve was successful because he was not trying to relax.

One constantly finds people who try to force themselves to fall asleep because they have read somewhere that it is dangerous if one doesn't sleep a certain specified amount. Trying to fall asleep, people become anxious and tense, and this, of course, makes the effort to sleep self-defeating. Only when they start trying hard to stay awake, to keep their eyes open, then, of course, they quickly fall asleep. This is what I call *paradoxical intention*, a phenomenon that on occasion makes for certain very effective forms of treatment. One German doctor in a sanitarium devoted to treating insomniacs simply ordered the patients to punch a time clock every quarter of an hour. After three-quarters of an hour everyone was fast asleep!

"Enjoy yourself and be happy!" At the risk of contradicting a paragraph of the Declaration of Independence, I must say that the "pursuit of happiness" is self-defeating. For it is the very pursuit that thwarts happiness. This can be readily observed in cases of sexual neurosis. The more a man wishes to show how sexually potent he is, to that very extent he becomes impotent. The more a woman tries to demonstrate, even if only to herself, how capable she is of orgasm, the more she is likely to be frigid.

Man does not strive merely for pleasure but also for meaning. Man is self-transcending. He is searching for a cause to serve or a person to love. He is truly human only to the extent to which he overlooks and forgets, and then gives his own self.

What happens in sexual neurosis is what logotherapy terms "hyperintention"—a person striving hard to prove himself potent or capable of orgasm. And this is reinforced by what we call "hyperreflection": too much watching of oneself. In *Man's Search for Meaning*° I described a woman suffering from frigidity. She had been sexually abused by her own father at the age of eleven, and she then read a great deal of vulgarized psychoanalytic literature, which convinced her that the traumatic experience would someday take its toll by way of a severe sexual neurosis. Thus, she became totally frigid. After our initial meeting, I told her deliberately, "I must put you on a waiting list. In two months we'll discuss it. For the time being, don't bother to think of your problem during intercourse, your orgasm or nonorgasm; but only think of your partner." Of course, you know what happened. She did not return in two months, but in two days—and she was cured. Why? Instead of hyperreflection, instead of watching herself and thinking about her problems, she simply forgot herself. And instead of hyperintention, instead of frantically striving for orgasm, she just gave herself. This is self-transcendence.

Man is one whole unit, and what is true of his ontological foundations is also applicable to such down-to-earth problems as frigidity and orgasm. Self-transcendence is a therapeutic agent, but it is also much more. It was Albert Schweitzer who once said, "The only ones among you who will be really happy are those who have sought and found how to serve." This is exactly what I have been trying to convey.

Now, what is at the root of this manipulative approach, this commanding, demanding, and ordering? You always try to command someone to believe, to hope, or to love. Yet this triad, this religious triad of faith, hope, and love, eludes any manipulative approach. This also holds for the will to meaning. You cannot command yourself or anyone to "have a will to meaning." If you wish to elicit the will to meaning in another

° Beacon Press, Boston, 1963.

person, you have to elucidate meaning itself in his presence. If this is done well, and it can be done well, then the will to meaning is automatically evoked in the human being sitting across from you.

I command you to laugh, but you cannot laugh simply at my command. If I want you to laugh, I have to tell you a joke. And this means we can only laugh *about* something. And that which we are laughing about, this person whom we are loving, that which we are hoping for, that being in whom we believe—these are intentional referents in the traditional terminology of Edmund Husserl, Max Scheler, and Franz Brentano, who founded the phenomenological movement three-quarters of a century ago.

This intentionality of mental activity in man is a reflection of what I have called, in more ontological terms, "the self-transcendent quality of human reality." But by manipulation you only succeed in shutting this quality out. For if you attempt to manipulate happiness or orgasm or potency or faith, you are inevitably objectifying, or reifying, them. But when you objectify a subject, a human person, when you try to turn him into an object, what is the result? Remember, the signal defining characteristic of a subject is that he has intentional acts, that he is directed toward intentional referents of his own. A subject is a subject only at the moment when he has objects of his own—which means when he is directed intentionally, self-transcendentally, toward a reality beyond himself. And to the very degree that you try to make a subject into an object, you are losing sight of his own objects, his own world. Thus, you are shutting out his intentionality and self-transcendence.

And, of course, this is applicable to the phenomenon of love. Jean-Paul Sartre defines love as a mutual process of making the other into an object. But this is most certainly not love. I prefer the definition, or better, the admonition, offered by another Frenchman, Antoine de St. Exupéry, who once said, "Love doesn't mean staring into one another's eyes, but love means looking in the same direction." Sartre's love is the staring into one another's eyes. Looking in the same direction, however, allows two people to remain subjects through a shared envisioning of meanings, values, and other beings. And this means that they can love.

Edith Weisskopf Joelson of the psychology department at the University of Georgia once did a statistical study, according to which the average American student is mostly interested in two things: self-interpretation and self-actualization. Now, self-actualization is not, and cannot become, an aim. Nothing would be more self-defeating. You may actualize yourself by fulfilling the meanings of your life or by giving yourself to another human being, but when you aim at self-actualization, you completely miss the mark. Abraham Maslow pointed out the same thing in his last writings.

But with regard to self-interpretation, the danger is hyper-reflection. If we dwell upon ourselves, watching ourselves, observing ourselves, contemplating ourselves, always focusing on ourselves, we are hyperreflecting ourselves and this is inevitably pathogenic. The famous philosopher Schelling said, "Pure reflection is the most dangerous disease of the human mind." And Goethe once said, "How is it that I've reached and achieved so much? Because I've never watched my own thinking. I've never thought about my thinking."

I have no objection to meditation. In fact, I have long pleaded for new forms of contemplative, meditative life to fill the increasing leisure hours created by industrialized society. But it must be meditation and contemplation without too much hyperreflection and, above all, with no hyperintention. It is self-defeating to try to grab hold of an experience in meditation or to prefabricate—or, should I say premeditate?—the form and content of meditation.

Consider this note, also from Edith Weisskopf Joelson: "I recently underwent some training in transcendental meditation. But I gave it up after a few weeks because I feel I meditate spontaneously on my own. When I start meditating formally, I actually stop meditating." This sums up everything I have been saying. Therefore, take heed. The old Latins used to say, *"Videant consules."* I think this warning holds true not only for politicians but also, especially here in California, for the various teachers and therapists, for the *counselors* who are attempting to help in man's search for meaning. *Videant consules:* Counselors, take heed!

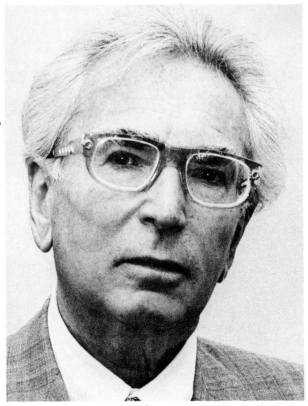

*Viktor E. Frankl, M.D., Ph.D.*, is Professor of Neurology and Psychiatry at the University of Vienna Medical School and Professor of Logotherapy at the United States International University in San Diego. He is the internationally renowned originator of the school of logotherapy and the author of *Man's Search for Meaning, The Doctor and the Soul, Psychotherapy and Existentialism*, and most recently published in English, *The Unconscious God.*

# THE RELATIONSHIP
# OF PSYCHOTHERAPY
# TO SACRED TRADITION

## A. C. Robin Skynner

I hope you will not mind if I speak rather personally. I am not a scholar—to my regret—but a craftsman of sorts, and I find even in the course of my professional teaching I communicate best when I speak from my own experience. It soon became clear to me that this was the only position from which I could approach the question we are examining here in this series and that I could only seek to live with the question more intensely than before, bringing it into contact with as much of my daily experience as possible and remaining attentive and open to the information it brought me. I have been made aware once again that this questioning attitude, and the immediate, receptive, and sensitive responsiveness to my life which it brings about, is perhaps the only useful answer to our question, if the idea of an "answer" is even appropriate at all. I therefore bring this attitude here and hope that some of you will share it with me.

This being so, perhaps I should begin by establishing my credentials, giving you some information about the path that has led me here so that you can better judge how much or how little you can trust what I have to say. Professor Needleman spoke of a Celtic fable in which two brothers pass each other on a mountain; one is being dragged down by a black dog to which he is attached by an iron chain, the other is being drawn up by a golden thread attached to a mysterious crane somewhere above. The story has enchanted and preoccupied me since, perhaps because I am a Celt myself—in fact, a Cornishman—and, as I expect you know, Celtic dogs of this particular breed are perhaps bigger, blacker, and more difficult to manage than most.

Certainly I was attracted to the study of psychiatry by a need to find a way of dealing with my own problems. And my present interest in training mental-health professionals leads me to believe that this is not only the usual motivation for taking up such work, consciously or unconsciously, but also the best one, provided it leads the professional to a real, direct, and systematic study of himself rather than a vicarious one through the study of his patients.

Without doubt, the knowledge I gained from my studies of psychotherapy provided some help in finding a different relationship to this unruly animal. Even before my own group analysis began, an attempt at self-analysis during my student days, based at first on the ideas of some of your so-called "neo-Freudians," particularly Horney, Fromm, and Sullivan, led the dog to begin a strange series of changes that have continued ever since. Though at first it took the form of quite severe depressive states coming "out of the blue," which formed part of a manic-depressive pattern common in my family, it soon changed to black rage, which in some ways was more difficult to deal with but at least began to be an understandable and a meaningful part of me. As the dog assumed forms related to ever-earlier periods of my life, something of great force and potential also became available, manifested by a sudden ability to learn and to work constructively, which has persisted since, a fairly complete disappearance of an incapacitating stutter which had until then made communication difficult, and the beginning of an ability to relate more simply and pleasurably with others. I mention this because ideas that can produce such effects must have some validity, and I feel it is important to add that these consequences seemed connected with a perception of the truth of many of the basic Freudian conceptions, particularly infantile sexuality and the Oedipus Complex, which led to a simple acceptance and enjoyment of ordinary sexuality not only in bed but also as this subtle energy pervades all relationships. I remember too the wonderful recognition that a strain of violence that had permeated my family history could be welcomed rather than escaped from, like a fearsome, untamed animal that could be a source of energy if one could find the right relationship to it.

At this time I was an agnostic, indeed a quite militant atheist writing regularly for the *Rationalist Annual*. But while still undergoing psychiatric training I took part with other students as a research subject in an investigation into the effects of LSD, which had just then become available in England. Some of my fellow students had fearful paranoid hallucinations that haunted them for some time afterward, but my own experience was more fortunate—a perception of successive, ascending levels of reality and consciousness, and of the interconnectedness and meaningfulness of everything, all of which I retained as a certainty afterward and which exactly coincided with descriptions of mystical experience and religious ecstasy I had previously brushed aside as fantasy. I saw that this was what I had been searching for all along. And though I realized that drugs could do no more than enable one to glimpse such possibilities, and therefore did not use this approach again, the experience led me to a deep and increasing interest in the relevance of sacred tradition.

My own analysis—a combination of group and individual—took place some time after this interest had developed, so that I had the experience—perhaps rather unusual—of being under the influence of sacred tradition and psychotherapy simultaneously. And, of course, I have been working as a psychotherapist with individuals, groups, families, and institutions ever since, while also continuing this guided search for the deeper, spiritual significance of my life. In this series of lectures I belong, then, among the psychotherapists rather than the spiritual guides—the "shrinks" rather than the "gurus."

Now what does a psychotherapist do? I don't mean *how* does he do it but rather *what* does he expect reliably to achieve, in the way, for example, that carpenters take it for granted that, given adequate wood, they can make a table that will not fall apart, or plumbers expect water to flow from taps they have installed. Such astonishing misconceptions surround this area, in my experience, that a few simple facts are necessary if we are to communicate at all. Professor Needleman has spoken of the recent overvaluation and current disillusionment with ordinary psychology and psychotherapy in the United States. In England we have perhaps been luckier, for psychoanalysis has never been taken very seriously there either by the general public or by the medical profession, least of all by orthodox psychiatry, where it has never enjoyed (or suffered from) the power and influence it until recently possessed in America. At the same time, it is true that some of its effects are almost as pervasive as they have been here: the idealization of infancy and the child/mother relationship, the cult of the individual, the belief in indulgence and self-expression, the devaluation of the role of the father and of authority, structure, and discipline in family and social life generally.

This is not to say that psychiatrists are not assumed to see right through people and to be secretly analyzing them at parties, when they are in fact only trying to attract the attention of the waiter, like everybody else. But I fancy that this overvaluation, even in the United States, is always accompanied by the other side of the coin, a complete disbelief that a psychotherapist can do anything at all except listen to rich old ladies and pocket their savings. Certainly I am constantly made aware, especially by acquaintances following one or another of the traditional paths, that though they accept that we might be able to relieve discomfort by drugs and soothing falsehoods, we could not possibly achieve much in the way of reliably facilitating change in those who come to see us. This is nonsense, of course, as untrue as the obverse assumption that we can change the world.

Because psychotherapy means so many things, I am going to stick to one or two brief examples, which can sometimes convey more than generalizations. The day Professor Needleman's essay arrived I found beside it in my letter rack three Christmas cards from ex-patients. One would be rather worried if one received many such messages, for in the better therapeutic results people are too busy leading full lives and enjoying real relationships to maintain contact with the therapist, even though some warmth and gratitude usually remain. Typically they say, if you bump into them in the street, "I've been meaning to write for years, but I never seem to get around to it." But one does get a few communications, especially a brief note with a Christmas card after a year or two, and of course it is very pleasant to hear how things are going.

The first was from a business executive who throughout his life was childish, violent, and destructive in any close relationship with a woman, accompanied by bouts of alcoholism. He had left therapy at a point where the drinking was under control and he had sustained a relationship with a woman long enough to plan to marry her. In his card he said things were going very well. And the goal of marriage, which was his main hope, was evidently achieved, for he signed his card from his wife as well as himself.

The second card was from Australia, from a doctor's wife whose profoundly disturbed relationship with her mother had led to an inability to love her daughter and to sexual frigidity after the child arrived, as well as to chronic depression and other marital problems. After confirming that improvements in those areas had been maintained, she concluded: "I think leaving the group has been awfully good for me as I have had to fend for myself and with the three years I'd had with you all—although it's been tough—the 'end' result is a very happy one. I feel alive and indestructible! I think of you all often and very fondly."

The third was from a couple living abroad in Europe, who had flown across for a few sessions because of a pathological sexual jealousy on the wife's part, really at a psychotic level and based on her fantasy but fed nevertheless by the husband's weakness and nervous secretiveness. The task with them was to help the husband maintain his identity against his wife's implacable, devouring possessiveness, and it seems that something had in fact improved, even though the form the message took was another manifestation of the problem. Clipped to the Christmas card, which was signed by them both, was a blank piece of paper saying "very much improved" followed by the husband's initials. (Her delusions included the idea that he was constantly sending secret messages!)

I will add a fourth which arrived two months earlier and which I found when I put the cards away. This was from a young married woman lacking any secure sense of identity and so unable to control her intense negative feelings that I had found it difficult to be in the same room with her and would not have taken her on for therapy myself had she not been so persistent in seeking it. As so often happens with such cases, she worked hard and did unusually well over her year of attendance, and sent a card some months later from Los Angeles, to where she had returned. I will quote this in more detail, because it conveys so well what the psychotherapeutic process meant to her:

> I guess the most important thing to say is that what I gained from being with you all is extremely supportive during a period of enormous adjustment. I truly carry you all around with me—and am able to accept the ups and downs with much more equanimity and lack of self-doubt than before. It is possible now to be more open and honest, without being consumed and defeated by self-doubt. I think I will never lead a conventional life, but I am better able now to contain that reality and not be so frightened and disturbed by it [I think this is a reference to her

bisexuality], even to enjoy its good side. I send you all much love and all best wishes for continued progress and support—the same which enabled me to take hold of my own life and not feel so helpless in doing so.

All these people, you will notice, had failed to develop an adequate sense of identity (in Erikson's sense), having failed to internalize in their early family environments adequate "models" of behavior and relationship, which could subsequently serve as reliable guides to action. Change appeared to take place through increased awareness of the existing, inappropriate "models," accompanied by learning of new ones from the therapist or other group members—a kind of second, corrective family experience. This is made very clear by the note from the last patient mentioned, when she says, "I truly carry you all around with me. . . ."

Now none of these people displayed during their therapy any real interest in the deeper meaning of their life on this planet, orbiting our sun within its galaxy in this universe, at this time in its history. Usually I am given early on a clear indication from those patients who will later seek out a spiritual path. They are in some way more open and vulnerable, more aware of themselves as part of mankind, part of the universe, "leaves on a tree." They are more troubled about and interested in the meaning of their existence as a whole rather than the meaning of what happened to them yesterday or in their childhood, or in the hopes and fears of what will happen to them tomorrow. They behave as if they have at some time been given a view from higher up the mountain, which they dimly remember and which leads them thereafter to seek again what they once glimpsed. Such patients are more widely interested and more interesting to treat, not least because they are more directly challenging both to me as a person and to my practice as a psychotherapist. To work with them is a shared endeavor in which I am more in question and receive more myself in consequence.

At some point, often late in therapy, they usually express their impression that I am holding something back from them, that I have another kind of understanding, which is implicit in all I do and say but not directly communicated. (This never happens with the other patients.) At this point I may become more explicit, though always in the context of the therapy, which remains my central concern, and within the context also of what they already understand. Some, previously members of established churches, may eventually return again to their faith with a more mature relationship to it, often after an earlier period in the therapy when they have rejected religion, or rather rejected the childish, magical attitude toward it with which they came. Others find their way to the Eastern teachings, which have emerged in England as here—some, for example, without any suggestion from me went to a Tibetan Buddhist monastery in Scotland.

This is not to say that other patients, or at least those whose treatment is successful, do not develop a deeper sense of themselves as part of something larger. Such a loss of egocentricity is, as Alfred Adler insisted, an inevitable accompaniment of any improvement, perhaps the most fundamental change of all. But there has always been for me a clear distinction between these patients and those who cannot forget that they have once perceived this other meaning of life, who behave as if they are in some way "children of God."

Now why is it that these two kinds of inquiry are confused at all? Perhaps we could look first at features that *appear* similar between them, which might lead to some confusion.

First of all, there is in both psychotherapy and tradition the idea that man's perception is clouded and distorted—that he does not see things as they are but as he wants to see them. In the spiritual teachings there are the ideas of samsara, the false world of appearances, the shadows in Plato's cave; in psychotherapy we have the defenses of denial, projection, idealization, and withdrawal into fantasy.

Second, in both, man is seen as being divided. His problems and suffering are believed to stem from this fragmentation, this failure to become whole and to take responsibility for himself.

Third, self knowledge, whereby he can find the lost parts of himself and become whole again, is seen as the key to the rediscovery of his integrity, so that he may become no longer divided into "I" and "not-I"—identifying himself with some parts of his being and rejecting others, which then become projected and perceived in negative fashion in those around him.

Fourth, this rediscovery and reacceptance is in both processes expected to be painful but regarded as bitter medicine that can ultimately heal and lead to growth. In individual and group psychotherapy, in encounter techniques, in the Synanon "haircut," and in the challenging confrontations of family and marital therapy, we find a systematic exposure of associations of thought, or of spontaneous emotional responses, or of actions, in a situation where, though it is supportive and containing, escape is prevented and the truth has sooner or later to be acknowledged. In the "confession of sins," in the acceptance of whatever internal manifestations arise during the stillness of meditation, in the openness to the inner voice of conscience, which is sought during the concentration of prayer, similar processes appear to be occurring. The unconscious is made conscious, the self is expanded as denial and projection are reduced and dissociated parts return; the lost sheep is found, the prodigal returns and is welcomed. Following from this, in both tradition and in psychotherapy a clearer perception of the world and a greater capacity to understand, accept, and relate to others can be seen to follow from this greater self-acceptance and objectivity.

Fifth, both see man as possessing hidden resources, which cannot become available without this greater self knowledge

A REVIEW COPY FROM
## Alfred · A · Knopf

WE WOULD APPRECIATE RECEIVING
TWO COPIES OF YOUR REVIEW.

TITLE:   ON THE WAY TO SELF KNOWLEDGE
AUTHOR:  NEEDLEMAN & LEWIS EDS.
PRICE:   $8.95
PUB DATE: OCTOBER 15 1976

PLEASE DO NOT RUN YOUR REVIEW
BEFORE PUBLICATION DATE.

and integration, even though the scale of this hidden potential is differently perceived in different schools of psychotherapy and, of course, even more so between psychotherapy generally and the spiritual traditions.

Sixth, as a corollary, much of man's suffering and pain is in both regarded as unnecessary, a product of ignorance and blindness, of confusion and complexity resulting from the inner division and the deceit and subterfuge necessary to preserve some illusion of coherence: intellectualization, fantasy, Jung's "persona," the "ego" in the ordinary sense, Horney's "ideal image," and what Krishnamurti calls "thought." It is expected, therefore (and it is the case), that negative feelings, suffering, and pain (or at least those which serve no useful purpose) gradually diminish and disappear in the course both of competent psychotherapy and the following of a sacred tradition.

And finally, seventh, both require that the searcher shall be in personal, regular contact with a teacher, guide, guru, analyst, or leader who has already been through the same experiences; has seen, understood, and accepted at least some aspects of himself; has escaped from some of his own fragmentation, delusions, and distorted perceptions; and so can, through being able to perceive the searcher more objectively, help him in turn to become more objective about himself.


There is, as we see, much *apparent* overlap, and I think we may be forgiven if we experience some confusion, at least initially, between these different kinds of exploration. My personal experience leads me to believe, however, that these two paths lie, if not in opposite directions, at least in quite different dimensions, and that we need to look for a much more subtle relationship between them. The fable of the two brothers, the golden thread, and the black dog, and the idea of the third brother arising from the relation between them, hints at this. Having looked at some similarities between these two paths, let us now summarize some of the differences, which I believe are not only greater but incommensurately greater.

First, all sacred traditions begin from the idea of an ordered, intelligent universe, where the idea of *hierarchy* is central and where each level is related to others in reciprocal dependence. Man appears very low down on this scale of being, though he has a definite place and serves purposes beyond himself, necessary to the total structure.

Second, in the sacred traditions man is perceived as having a choice of two purposes he may serve in this grand design— God or Caesar; the ordinary world of appearances or a more real world behind it; his natural appetites and desires or an inner voice or conscience, which comes into conflict with these; the black dog, perhaps, or the golden thread. The traditions tell us that we all serve nature, in our ordinary state of development, as unconsciously as the grass feeds the cow and its manure in turn feeds the grass again; and that our illusion of power and freedom, and our fantasies about ourselves and mankind, ensure that we do this, just as the beast of burden walking endlessly in a circle to drive the primitive pump is kept at its job by the pole attached to its back and the blindfold that prevents it from seeing its true plight. But the traditions tell us that it is also possible, in the scheme of things, for some men to awaken to the situation and to perceive another possibility, another task they can fulfill, another influence that, if they can submit to it, will free them in some measure from the blindness and slavery of their ordinary existence. Though they must still live on earth, a connection begins to be made with heaven. For the person who is awakened to this other realm, a higher energy, a more subtle intelligence becomes available and begins to change the whole purpose and meaning of ordinary life, though the latter continues as before and may show little change of a kind discernible to those still circling the treadmill and absorbed in their dreams. Caesar must still be served, but the service of God transforms this totally and causes life to become an endlessly rich source of knowledge and experience to feed the new life growing like a child within the person called to this new service.

Now this kind of idea is not part of ordinary psychology, whether "scientific" or "humanistic." Though the latter might recognize and show more serious interest in some of the *experiences* previously called "religious" or "mystical," man is still perceived as being at the center of things; his ordinary desires, ambitions, hopes, and plans, whether selfish or altruistic, are taken at face value and used as a basis for action, for planning utopias and eupsychias. There is no concept of the second purpose to which man can give himself, and because of this, no real questioning whether the first could be illusory. Ordinary psychology then becomes another elaboration of the delusion itself, providing more blindfolds, another ring through the nose, more "hope" to keep us turning the treadmill.

Third, and following on from this, the possibility of recognizing and beginning to understand the significance of the sacred traditions begins from a disillusionment with ordinary life, with one's ordinary self, with ordinary knowledge. Only after the blindfold is removed and we see we are going in a circle all the time have we the hope of choosing another direction. We have to see that life is not going anywhere in the way we formerly imagined, that it never has and never will. Having faced this, we may realize that no escape is possible from the repetition of our ordinary level without help from another. Coming to disbelieve in our ordinary thought and emotion, and so becoming still enough and open enough to reach a deeper and more fundamental part of ourselves where another energy, a different possibility of consciousness exists, a connection may be made, since we are for a moment available for it. Thus we have to begin from the point of failure, to relinquish our valuation of our ordinary selves and to let this be replaced gradually by something which at first does not seem to be ourselves at all. Having awakened, we have to die in order to be reborn.

Now does not ordinary psychology rather lead to an *increase* of our ordinary self, more efficient, more fruitful, more enjoyable, and less conflicted perhaps, but still the same thing writ larger, the same ambitions fulfilled instead of unfulfilled, the same desires satisfied instead of frustrated? Ordinary psychology surely seeks to *improve* the self, according to the ideas *of* the ordinary self; it scarcely seeks to destroy it.

Fourth, sacred traditions are by definition, if they are anything at all, a manifestation of the higher level about which they tell us, a point at which the levels actually touch each other. And, perhaps because they can only touch *within* man himself, they have been transmitted by a chain of individuals who actually manifest, with part of their being (rather than simply know about), the possibility with which these traditions are concerned. From this follow two further differences between the paths. One is the idea that the traditions have always existed, from the beginning of recorded time, and are simply spread into the world from the human chain that transmits them, the influence widening or contracting from one period to another and the means of expression being adapted to the prevailing forms of thought and current ordinary knowledge, though always conveying the same essential truth. If anything, the understanding *deteriorates* as it spreads wider from the teachers, like ripples on a pond. This is totally different from ordinary psychology, where knowledge is seen as a progressive development beginning perhaps from Mesmer and the nineteenth-century hypnotists, and leading through the pioneering work of Janet, Freud, Adler, and Jung to the achievements of the present day. For ordinary psychology, the present time is one of unusual enlightenment and progress; for the sacred traditions, it is more likely to be seen as a dark age.

A fifth difference, which also follows from what was just said, concerns the relationship between teacher and pupil. The ordinary psychotherapist would certainly recognize a difference in authority between himself and his patient based on age, experience, knowledge, and skill, but this would be expected to change in the course of treatment. As the patient matures, it is hoped that the "transference" is dissipated, and, while some regard and gratitude may remain, persistent dependency and acceptance of the analyst's authority are taken correctly to indicate incomplete treatment. In the sacred traditions, by contrast, the teacher is in some part of his being an actual manifestation of a higher level, and so a sharply hierarchical pupil/teacher relationship is not only appropriate but, since the human chain continues presumably all the way up the mountain, the authority of the guide, or of the next man above on the rope, may appropriately continue indefinitely. (I am less sure about this difference than about the others. Though essentially true, I think analogous developmental processes must nevertheless occur in both kinds of change.)

I will mention other differences more briefly. The most important is the different view of consciousness, already clearly expressed by Professor Needleman. Following what one might call an "archaeological" concept of consciousness, our ordinary Western psychology tends to assume that we already possess the light of consciousness but that some parts of ourselves have been buried and need to be found and brought into this light again, after which they will remain at least potentially accessible. The light is assumed to be burning already, at least while we are out of bed and moving about, and its brightness and continuity are not very much questioned. By contrast, the great traditions maintain explicitly or implicitly the idea that man's consciousness is much more limited, fluctuating, and illusory than he usually realizes, and that an extraordinary amount of persistent effort is needed even to maintain it more steadily, let alone increase it. For the traditions, consciousness is more like the light powered by a dynamo, driven by the wheel of a bicycle, where we have to pedal constantly if it is to remain alight and pedal harder to make it brighter. It is true, of course, that the idea that attention and consciousness require effort and work, as well as the idea of finer levels of energy generated by the effort of more sustained attention, and the further idea that the two can lead automatically to the reintegration of dissociated psychic elements, are all present in the ideas of Janet, the Frenchman who in so many ways anticipated Freud. But then Janet was a religious man, and his eclipse by Freud was no doubt another consequence of the attitudes current in this epoch.

If we are to accept these differences as valid, it seems to me that they lead us to a view of psychotherapy and of sacred tradition as different dimensions at right angles to each other, with fundamental aims that cannot in their nature coincide at all. Psychotherapy is about ordinary life, the development of man along the horizontal line of time from birth to death. Just as the physician is concerned with countering threats to life and obstacles to physical growth, and remedying deficiencies and deviations in the development of the body, so the function of the psychotherapist (which developed originally, and is still based most firmly, within the role of the physician) can be seen as averting threats to psychological stability, relieving obstacles and inhibitions in the process of growth from the dependency of the child to the relative responsibility and autonomy of the adult. To do so the psychotherapist seeks to supply those experiences that have been lacking in the patient's history, particularly those that were missing or distorted in the early family environment.

The sacred traditions begin from the horizontal line of time but are concerned with a quite different, vertical line of development: man's increasing awareness of, connection with, and service to the chain of reciprocal transformation and exchange among levels of excellence, which the cosmic design appears to need some (but not all or even most) of mankind to fulfill. There is an analogy here with the physical sphere, where man is obliged to move about on the horizontal, two-dimensional surface of the earth if he is to survive at all but is not obliged to fly and exist in the three-dimensional atmosphere, though he can do so if he wishes and may find that this has consequences for his ordinary existence.

If these two endeavors are in fact quite distinct, then forms of psychotherapy that confuse them could be much more harmful to the possibility of spiritual development than those that do not recognize the existence of the traditions at all. Thus I believe that the ideas offered by such people as Maslow, Fromm, Rogers, and many leaders of the encounter movement may as easily hinder as help people toward a recognition of their actual position. It is true that these approaches may indeed stimulate a desire for the kind of understanding that only the traditions can supply, and I am grateful for the way in which they have all personally assisted me. But because they mix the levels, they stand in danger of offering a half-truth sufficiently like the real thing to satisfy this deeper hunger without leading to anything more real and even, as Needleman has suggested, of simply increasing the attachment to the ordinary self. Jung, too, though so much admired by people of a religious persuasion, in contrast to that terrible Sigmund Freud, seems to me to offer a particularly subtle temptation, precisely because of the depth and quality of his personal understanding, together with his fundamental confusion of psychology and sacred tradition, psyche and spirit.

This is why when I cannot find a good eclectic psychotherapist (in the sense of someone who seeks to integrate the best of the different schools) I tend to refer patients to competent Freudian analysts, provided they are agnostic rather than militantly atheistic and demonstrate by the quality of their lives that they are decent and responsible people. For I find that the better Freudians at least have their feet on the ground rather than their heads in the clouds, a good beginning if one wishes to travel reliably along the surface of the earth. Being concerned first and foremost with the development of ordinary competence in making a living, forming responsible relationships, enjoying sexuality and other natural appetites, raising a family, and generally coping adequately with life, they help to establish a firm base from which an interest in deeper meaning can develop.

The differences now seem clear enough, and it is hard to see how we could ever confuse these two different kinds of development. At this point we can all feel satisfied. Followers of sacred traditions can reassure themselves that, after all, they did not really need to have that analysis which seemed so much to improve the life of their neighbor. The psychotherapist can also feel relieved, finally satisfied that people who follow a traditional path are not really living in the real world and are best left to their delusions. I can comfort myself that I have answered in some measure the question Professor Needleman set us in his introductory talk. Had I been wiser, I would have arranged matters so that I could stop here and be well on my way home before the cracks appear and the whole edifice falls to pieces.

But if we go on, I fear that the simplicity disappears. Even though I believe that what I have said is correct as far as it goes, we begin to see that the important issue for us is the relationship that exists at the meeting point of these two dimensions: that cross, within each man, of the line of time and the line of eternity, level, or scale. In approaching this, I find I have to reconcile a number of facts, or at least a number of observations that I can no longer doubt.

The first is that many who follow a sacred tradition change profoundly as regards their ordinary life adjustment, whereby many of the problems that might otherwise take them to a psychotherapist simply melt away—like ice in the sun, disappearing without any systematic attempt to change—under the influence of some subtler, finer influence that begins to permeate and alter the whole organism.

Second, I have noticed that others who follow such traditions appear to become more closed, narrow, and intolerant both of others and of their own hidden aspects. Of those I see professionally, this group is the most intractable and untreatable of all, for the knowledge derived from a religious tradition has been put to the service of perceptual defense, of complacency, of narcissistic self-satisfaction, of comfort and security.

Third, the difficulties of working with such individuals are only equaled by those encountered with people who have misused the ideas and techniques of psychotherapy in a similar fashion. Excepting only the group that I have just mentioned, no patients are as difficult to treat as psychoanalysts, particularly those who believe they have had a "full analysis" (what a marvelous expression!) already.

And fourth, others in psychotherapy, particularly those in psychotherapy groups, and almost routinely those at a certain stage in large groups run in the way we attempt it in London—and I think also in encounter groups in the early stages, before they become a new game—can reach a point of simple openness, of awareness of themselves as part of mankind and of the universe, and of direct communion with others, more intensely than many following a traditional teaching, at least as far as one can judge from the statements and external behavior of each. It does not last, of course, and cannot be pursued systematically, but in the psychotherapeutic experience it is often there, sometimes in an awe-inspiring fashion, and we have to make a place for this in our ideas.

For some time after writing this I was uncomfortable with it and could take it no further, till I saw that I had assumed, for want of any real question to myself, that I might belong to the first or fourth groups but that the second and third were made up of other people. But a moment's reflection showed that I was a member of all four, and that the principal obstacles to my own development were precisely those that stemmed from the misuse of such professional or religious understanding as I possessed, in order to preserve and enhance my ordinary image of myself. And this, I see, applies to us all; it is in the nature of things.

Whether in my ordinary life or in my search for its hidden significance, I am most alive, closest to the source and meaning of my existence, when I am open to my immediate experience, receptive to what it can teach me and vulnerable to its power to change my being. In this moment, when I am sure of nothing, I am yet most deeply confident of the possibility of understanding. My actions spring most truly from myself, yet I have no idea beforehand what I will manifest. Like water welling up from a spring, I am new every moment, appearing miraculously from some source hidden deep within the ground of my being.

The next instant I have lost this movement, this freedom, this life constantly renewed, and am once again trying to be right, to be good, to know, to change, to be normal, to be successful—or alternatively to be bad, rebellious, a tragic failure, a pathetic victim—but one way or another always seeking to preserve some experience, like a butterfly gassed in a bottle and pinned to a board, losing in the process everything that made me wish to capture it in the first place. Seeking security, certainty, and beliefs to buoy me up, I cling to my experience in order to preserve it, but find myself holding only the dead residue of a living process that has already changed and moved elsewhere. Small wonder that I find my life colorless, dull, flat, and boring, needing ever-increasing artificial stimulation to restore me to some feeling of alertness.

Perceiving this, I realize that I must live nearer the source of this inner spring, somehow maintaining myself at the point where this "living water" gushes forth into the visible world. I may see that I am constantly carried by the current into the more superficial manifestations to which this energy gives rise as it flows away from the source, that it cannot be different while I remain passive, my attention captured and carried downstream by the flow. Once I see this, I may begin to swim against the current, struggling to remain closer to the source, where my life is constantly renewed, no longer trying to hold on to things for fear of sinking, and realizing that the formlessness and endless change from which I shrink is a condition of real life itself.

If I can only realize my true situation and thereby loosen my attachment to the forms my life energy takes as it moves further from its origin, I may find that I *remember* the source, and that this memory brings a desire to find it again. Now I find myself swimming against the current to regain it, from love and delight; the effort follows directly from my desire, just as my heart beats faster as I begin to run, and my running follows from my perception of the goal I wish to reach. I need only free myself from my hypnosis long enough to remember what I have lost.

Then I am in the middle, between the hidden source of my life in a higher realm and its manifestations in this world, and I must then struggle not to deny either. If I forget the source, I drift downstream toward increasing repetition; or if I forget the nature of the stream itself and its constant downward pull, then I begin to dream I am already at the source, rather than to experience it and to swim toward it, and so I drift downstream again. Only when I realize my nature as a creature of two worlds do I discover the full potential of my life, which must be lived everlastingly between them.

Now this immediate experience of my living energy can be brought about by many kinds of events. Vivid and profound emotional experience can produce it, such as death of a loved one, the birth of a child, sometimes sexual love, great beauty, pain, an event on a world scale. Drugs like LSD and mescaline can give a taste of such experience by their capacity to destroy defenses and release emotion, and so can psychotherapy, particularly perhaps encounter techniques and the gestalt approaches that seek to release the most primitive and childlike emotions.

But without deeper knowledge we drift downstream imagining we still live at this zenith, while the experience in fact becomes degraded, copied and repeated, fantasized. Then we need larger doses, stronger stimuli, bigger groups, new techniques to startle us out of our dreams again. If this is in fact the case, it would at least explain why those undergoing analysis appear for a time more real and open, only to become more closed than others sometimes, when the analytic process is over, particularly if there is a professional vested interest in demonstrating a good result. Many will recognize exactly the same process among followers of the sacred traditions—a marvelous openness and simplicity in younger people just beginning, deteriorating gradually toward complacency, rigidity, and parroting of formulas in those who begin to "know" and, in doing so, cease to live.

It is here, perhaps, that the place of the family and community as a "middle zone," and the need for ordinary effort and work, become vital factors, as Needleman has emphasized. For our natural tendency to drift with the streaming of our life energy into increasingly dead and ritualized manifestation—or to put it another way, our predisposition to convert real experience into fantasy and then repeat it, so that our lives not only become B-movies but even the same old B-movie over and over again—is so great that we need the discipline of *effort* to convince us, through our constantly experienced inability to swim against *any* current, that we are always drifting. And for this we need also the discipline of a group of intimates who know us well and love us enough to make demands on us for ordinary effort, who remind us when we drift too far from our more real selves and begin to live in dreams and selfish fantasies, and who demand of us that we be not less than ordinary men and women, fulfilling our ordinary responsibilities. For if we are not at least this, how can we hope to be more? Here, I believe, psychotherapy has its proper place, above all in the facilitation of this function of the family and the outer discipline and support it provides, or the provision of substitute group experience where this is missing. Given this ground, the sacred traditions have some possibility to guide us back to the source of our lives.

# A. C. Robin Skynner: *Questions*

*Question:* Would you expand a little on this business of wanting to be right? In my experience with the ways of tradition, it's appropriate to laugh at people who have a strong impulse to be right. But it seems to me that one is not really biting the bullet, because when those same people who feel it appropriate to laugh are up in an airplane, they seem to hope that the pilot has a sufficiently strong impulse to be right. Competency is expected in certain technical affairs on this terribly ordinary, miserable, mundane level, especially when life or money is involved. But on the "higher" level one is always urged to "give up" and face the unknown and realize that you don't understand. But if I were an employer, I wouldn't want to employ people who didn't understand—who didn't know what they ought to know. They would quickly get the sack. And yet there's often a kind of cop-out with people in the religious realm, a belief that their mistakes are reversible, since neither they nor anyone else will be harmed as a result. But obviously something must be at stake. There must be some responsibility. And it seems to me that when you sense your responsibility there's a real tension between the incredible importance of not being wrong and the terrible limitations of wishing to be right. Would you care to expand on that?

*Dr. Skynner:* Well, I can try. Certainly, having flown six thousand miles here and having to fly six thousand back, I feel entirely sympathetic toward the pilot and plane builder who want to be right. But taking myself as an example, I can tell you what took place in front of the challenge to think about the relationship between psychotherapy and the sacred. I had always kept them in rather different compartments and more or less hoped that they would sort things out between themselves when I wasn't looking. And so it was very good to have to come here and speak about them, to have to actually

226

live with this question and try to put it down on paper. What I found was that I couldn't "get it right." Every time I thought I had got the relationship right, it all turned upside-down and I had to start again. At first the relationship seems somewhat similar, then totally different, then in fact it's more complicated. And I think the only answer I can give to your question has to do with training people in group psychotherapy, where I come up against this issue more often than in other situations. When you work with a group you somehow have to be able to feel with the group but not lose your wits; that is, you have to use your *mind* at the same time that you are *feeling* with the others. One tends to escape into thinking, which is easy, or just feeling, which is also easy. To have the two on at the same time is very difficult. If in fact we start to conceptualize our experience and try to "get" it right, we end up with something we can use in certain ways, but it's dead—we've killed it. It's like the butterfly on the board. You can study it in a way that you can't when it's flying, but you have killed it. And I think we have to find our way between these two experiences. We have to have both things, both possibilities, there. But for this I think we have to leave things behind all the time. When we do conceptualize, we then have to move on and begin to be open to newer experience. It's really just a description of scientific method, when you think about it.

*Same questioner:* Well, I think there's a danger there. In a scientific crisis, everything may have to be reworked from the ground up, but you still have to retain a lot of the knowledge that has been won from the past. Any new reworking that cannot include those old things is no good. So it's not just that people have to start again, and do it all again—it doesn't mean that they haven't got even more constraints than they had in the past.

*Answer:* I think it has something to do with the way we *use* our knowledge. As long as we actually use it for some practical purpose, that's fine—because we're willing to lose it, or to change it, or to be open to new experience that makes it different. But I think the danger comes when we begin to hang on to it, and cling to it—like we cling to a life raft—and then we're not open to new experience; we're just stuck. But I think it's possible to be totally open and at the same time to be aware, in the present moment, of what you already know. Does anyone else have any ideas on this?

*Question:* I have a different question. You talked about the similarities between psychotherapy and sacred tradition, and you also talked about the differences. But what about a person who is in therapy and is *also* following a tradition? . . .

*Answer:* Well, I think they can help each other enormously, provided there's a right relationship between them. My experience is of being pulled in two opposite directions and of the tension that results being helpful to both. In talking to other people in the same situation, it's clear they've had the same kind of experience. Certainly these two approaches are not incompatible.

*Same questioner:* Could you say something about how you go about finding the right relationship?

*Answer:* I think you have to be open to both. The difficulty is that we always hedge our bets. Often when we do both at once, we use one to avoid the other. This is why it's probably sometimes better not to do both at the same time. Another problem is that we take some things to one place and other things to another place, but we never take the right things to the right place. But if in fact we can be more honest about it and try to play the game straight, then it's probably all right to be involved in both. But this means we must take ourselves fully to both situations, without saying "this belongs here and that belongs there," and we must accept what comes back to us. If we tell ourselves that psychotherapy is the right place to take our sex life, and sacred tradition is the right place to take our wish to be unified with God, then we are simply split down the middle and nothing will change.

*Question:* I am interested in asking about the unknown, the situation in which a person wants to find himself and reaches the point of *not knowing*—not knowing anything. He goes through many different kinds of experiences in trying to find an answer to his life, but now he comes to you and simply does not know. He has come to the end of the line. When you come to the end of the line where everything you've tried hasn't worked and you need guidance, must one then accept whatever guidance one finds? Have you ever dealt with people in such a situation? People who can more or less function in their lives—they can get that far—but they *don't know?* How are *you* able to be in that situation with someone who doesn't know, but who is there, there in front of you?

*Answer:* You just have to be fully there—that's all you can do. You can be there as yourself. I think that you can accompany people and keep them company in that state of not knowing. It's very difficult, and very frightening, and very painful not to know. But it's only out of that situation that knowledge or understanding comes—if you can bear it. That's my experience in psychotherapy. But most of the time we can't bear it and we latch on to something to feel more secure. But if one is with someone else or with a group of people who can support you in not knowing, then that not knowing can lead on to some real experience that you can perhaps trust more. In psychotherapy, at least in my experience, the main problem that keeps people from doing good work is that they want to help people. But once they begin to give up trying to help people and feeling they have to get good results, then something quite different begins to happen—some real communication begins to take place. But you can only be there in front of other people.

You're not satisfied?

*Same questioner:* I hear what you're saying.

*Question:* I think there are some terms in Western psychiatry that are very useful: for example, "regression in the service of the ego," "stages of cognitive development," "identity formation." Western psychiatry helps a person achieve all three of these things. Then they can begin to let go in a constructive way. But were you intimating in your talk that humanistic psychology tends to lock a person in his own ego structure and that this represents a danger?

*Answer:* I think the danger lies in a confusion of the different levels that one can feel. One believes that one is following the same sort of path and having the same sort of experiences as one does when following a religious discipline. But this just isn't so.

*Question:* You spoke about people entering a therapeutic process and then, later, of "graduating" into a spiritual tradition. Have you had experience with people who've done the reverse? For example, people who had been monks in Tibet, and found they'd gotten in over their heads and decided that perhaps psychotherapy was what they needed?

*Answer:* Yes, I have had experience of that. As I said before, there are many different sorts of people who come to psychotherapy. Working with those who use their religious beliefs as a defense, who hold on to them in order to maintain their existing personality structure, is very difficult because you're working against a very powerful adversary. But on the other hand, people who have had a very crucial relationship to a sacred tradition, who have practiced and worked within the tradition but have gotten stuck in some way, seem to do very much better and can use psychotherapy very much more quickly than people who haven't had that kind of practice. One of the things I have been struck by is that any technique which can be used for change and growth can also be used to stop it. The more powerful a technique is, the more dangerous it can be in preventing real change, if it is misused. That is why, I think, one shouldn't use these techniques on one's own. Whether in psychotherapy or in the spiritual search, one needs to be with others in order to see what is actually taking place.

*Question:* I'm wondering how you can be involved in psychotherapy and a spiritual tradition at the same time. Therapy seems to involve a reforming or changing of the self that is dependent on a continuation of identification, whereas sacred tradition involves dropping that identification. So I don't understand.

*Answer:* I'm glad you asked that, because I think it's something that needs to be discussed. But I think it was spoken about by Tarthang Tulku when he pointed out, more or less, that you can't give up your self until you've got one! In other words, you have to have a certain strength in your feeling of ordinary self before you can begin to renounce it or go beyond it. This is certainly true in my experience, and this is where psychotherapy has its value. It may get you ready to be able to meditate or to pray and so on. In fact just before I left for the United States I spoke to a patient of mine in England who had been going to one of the Tibetan Buddhist centers in London and who had left it to come back to therapy with me. Allow me to read to you a transcript of the conversation we had about this.

Dr. S: Could you put into words what you said when I asked that question about the problem you had had with attempting to meditate. I didn't write it down and I can't remember the words you used.

*Miss X:* What I felt was this. In Buddhism you are invited to examine your concept of yourself—it means your role, your self. And I think that is not to be confused with your actual existential feeling of yourself. If you haven't got a feeling of self, the ordinary self, and you try to meditate, you go psychotic. In other words, you have to have a "psychoanalytic" self, a feeling of togetherness, in order to meditate and abandon self in the Buddhist sense. Otherwise you go to pieces.

*Dr. S:* Did you find that happened to you—were you threatened with something like that?

*Miss X:* I found I could only meditate constructively when I felt together. Now that I don't feel together, I can't do it, and I have seen a lot of people—well, not a lot of people but several people—go psychotic in the Meditation Center in Scotland. I think it was because they had no central core that they could hold on to. I mentioned to you this concept from somewhere in the field of meditation, of "centering," that you need to do before you begin to meditate.

*Dr. S:* What does that mean?

*Miss X:* I think it means somehow gathering yourself together.

That's what she said. And I feel that's right. In other words, it's kind of a two-stage process, if you like. One has to first be able to cope with ordinary life. Of course, I'm not saying one can't do two things together, maybe strengthen ourselves at the same time that we receive and try to follow some teaching.

*Question:* Perhaps this relates to what you just said, but at one point in response to a question here you said that you have to bring the whole of yourself to whatever is in front of you. It was a question about doing psychotherapy and following a sacred tradition at the same time. But what if your problem is that you can't bring the whole of yourself to anything, and that wherever you are, there's very little of yourself there?

*Answer:* I think that psychotherapy can be a very great help in that, if it's well conducted. Certainly without an ordinary sense of wholeness it's impossible even to begin to meditate or to follow a sacred tradition. I think one needs to begin to approach oneself in a very simple kind of way, to get one's ordinary self together.

*Question:* How do you feel about the mixture of psychotherapy and sacred tradition that often occurs today, where, for example, it's common for people with no training to meditate in order to function better, and at the same time to substitute psychiatric labels for a direct experience of themselves? What I'm wondering about is the mixture between the two that exists in the world today among people who are not necessarily following either. You mentioned previously that some of the techniques that are used are very powerful and can have either beneficial or harmful results. Since these techniques have become much more available to us today through books, lectures, and so on, is there not some danger for those who are caught in the middle—reading these books yet not necessarily following a teaching or under psychoanalysis?

*Answer:* I think one can't do these sorts of things on one's own, because one needs some kind of accurate feedback. One doesn't know oneself well enough to know if one's going in the right direction. Not clearly seeing the direction, one tends to trip oneself up by stepping on one's own bootlaces. Therefore I think that work with a group can be extremely valuable. One shares experiences and gets direct feedback on quite an ordinary level from people who have similar concerns.

*Question:* I think it's important to realize that intellectualizations of one's path, whether it be psychotherapeutic or sacred, may in fact be a blockage of that path.

*Answer:* Yes, I agree with that. My experience has shown me that the value of psychotherapy isn't really in remembering the past but rather in seeing oneself over a long period of time, in perceiving oneself in the larger context of one's life. There is something curative in this that helps one become more objective toward oneself in the immediate present, which is what we talked about in the beginning.

*Question:* How do you use the ideas that you find in sacred traditions to help in the psychotherapeutic treatment of your patients—or do you?

*Answer:* I don't, at least not directly. The ideas affect the way I work, the way I *understand* what's happening. They help form some kind of ground on which I can operate. But I don't talk about it.

*Question:* There's a very generalized desire in me to work constructively together with other people—a desire, I suppose, that's at least partly due to the fact that I cannot work very long with myself. When I work with someone else, there can be a dialogue that opens me to new ways of looking. Now, when one is very young this wish for constructivity is met by something from other people that facilitates it. As soon as you try to take a step they encourage you to take the next step. But as one grows older that encouragement becomes a kind of opposition, and one soon develops one's own grating style on other people. I find for myself that this is a very important feature of the way I relate to other people. And I wish to find again that kind of working together that was natural when I was very young. When I was very young I used to speak with people, with adults, and there was a different relationship. They would *seriously* listen to what I had to say and try to draw out what my intention was. I would like very much to go back to that, to cooperate with people and have them recognize my special ability and give me enough space to use it in a way that gives me a feeling of full power. And of course I don't get that.

*Answer:* When one is a child, one is helped. One is taken by one's parents step by step; one is encouraged to go a bit further and is supported in each step one takes. And the whole thing is constructive; everyone is listening and working together. But you're saying that later on in life all this turns into opposition?

*Question:* Yes. When I was young, part of what I was interested in doing was helping people to approach things from a kind of simplicity and compassion. And this impressed many people because it was coming from the mouth of a very young child. Now, with only the memory of this simplicity in myself, I still see myself in that role, although it has changed because I've become clouded up and intoxicated with all kinds of opinions and ideas. So naturally people respond negatively. But I'm still trying to find that relationship.

*Answer:* Yes, I can understand that. The relationship you describe seems to me what a good psychotherapeutic relationship ought to be—a relationship in which one *is* listened to. This helps one to grow, to stretch a bit, to take the next step. But opposition is needed at some point. We need to struggle with somebody in order to discover our own real limits. So I think you have to go through these stages, both in psychotherapy and in childhood. But perhaps in the end one has to come to the end of all that and feel perhaps that despite having a lot of enjoyment, pleasure, or power in life, it's still empty—something is still missing. At that point I think one begins to look for some other means. And that's where the idea of sacred tradition comes in.

*Question:* Our culture seems to put a very high value on a certain kind of productivity, and as a result, the psychotherapy described is usually directed toward helping that productivity along—toward better social relations, becoming a good member of society, and so on. It strikes me that in some other more traditional cultures there was room for madness. And I'm wondering how sacred tradition—especially sacred traditions as they have operated in traditional societies—can bring psychotherapy the kind of attitude that would make it possible to listen to the mad, as it were.

*Answer:* This is quite important. Professor Needleman addressed this question at the beginning of the series when he spoke about earlier cultures, traditional cultures. If you were mad, you still had a place. It wasn't so long ago either. In the little village where I grew up, my father started a business and he employed the local village idiot, called Horace. He was not very intelligent, but he was as strong as a horse. And there was a place there for him, instead of his being shut away. Nowadays he would be in an institution. Unfortunately, we've lost the whole superstructure of understanding that can relate man to society in such a way that there *is* a place for everyone. We have to get back to that past, and psychotherapy does perhaps have to be brought together with these other, more traditional ideas. I don't know how to do it, but it has to be done.

*Question:* Could you speak about how techniques like free association and dream analysis correspond to similar techniques in the traditions? For instance, the effort to be present in the moment, that you spoke of, seems to contradict techniques like free association and dream analysis. I don't understand how those two different kinds of technique relate—whether it is possible to be present to oneself when one is imagining or dreaming, and what the value of that might be.

*Answer:* I think that free association may in fact give you a very startling sense of your own identity—briefly. And if that is what the chain of associations brings you, then the content isn't very important. In a sense you can throw it away—it's dead. You may, however, come across a thought or feeling that is quite unfamiliar to you and which may startle you into a new, wider interest in yourself. And the same is true for dreams. What seems important about dreams is that you carry them around with you and that you *feel* different the day afterward—you see things differently. The dream has altered your experience of yourself. That's probably more important than trying to understand it by cutting it up into bits.

*Question:* As a man who is mainly concerned with the vertical dimension in yourself—extraordinary ideas and so on—how is it possible to relate every day on a one-to-one basis with people who are primarily interested in ordinary things, patients to whom nothing is more important than being ordinary?

*Answer:* I'm not sure that I understand you.

*Same questioner:* In other words, you speak of therapy helping people on a horizontal plane, with their ordinary day-to-day lives. It would seem that many patients are voicing their impatience with themselves because they cannot deal with the day-to-day problems of living, and the most important thing to them would be to be able to deal with these problems. How can you, to whom that really is not the most important thing, work with these patients?

*Answer:* But it *is* the most important thing.

*Same questioner:* It is?

*Answer:* Yes. The only world is the world in front of one. But one is either there to experience it or one is not. And the sacred traditions are concerned with the question of whether we're actually close to this source of ourselves from which we can see everything anew—from which we can learn through a more direct interaction with the world. I don't see any contradiction at all, and I don't think there has to be. We can wake up to the fact that we have that possibility inside us. I was startled today, driving somewhere with Professor Needleman, when I saw the Pacific for the first time. I was quite astonished. I had heard about it all my life, but had never seen it. I can't remember exactly what I said, but perhaps Professor Needleman can.

*Dr. Needleman:* It was something like, "I must be here, because here I am!"

*Answer:* It was just a little thing, something that we have all experienced. The trouble is that this kind of perception is so simple that we cannot speak about it. Yet we have to speak about it, since it represents a different quality of receptivity— one that is our birthright.

*Question:* I see in people, as well as in myself, a deep irritation or a pain regarding both the past and the future. What I do not see, however, is how to measure or weigh the difference between that irritated or painful feeling that many of us carry around for a long time, and a feeling that might lead one to wish sincerely to change. Because for me, for anyone who wishes to change *now*, there doesn't seem to be anything available but time.

*Answer:* There are different ways of looking at that. One is that we have to accept the world as it is. I'm not saying we shouldn't have active functions in the world—things to do or to fulfill. But on a much larger scale, I think we have to accept that the world does work the way it does. Life is painful, and perhaps for a reason. Another point is that the more you work with people the more you see that there are very powerful forces holding us in our situation. And what's holding us usually is that we know how to do what we are doing. We've suffered all of our lives, we know what that's like. If we've had a nasty, bitchy, scolding mother, we know how to deal with that, and it's no surprise that we may find for a wife a woman who is also bitchy and scolding—partly because we know how to deal with it, partly because it feels like home, and partly because we *need* someone like that if we're going to get out of it. What I am saying is that our life as it is provides at least some of the conditions we need for an understanding that can transform us, that can free us from our dependency on what we "know" so well. This is something one sees in psychotherapy. But one has to accept that one can't do very much; one needs compassion. Then many things are possible. I think we underestimate, all the time, what other people are capable of. We always want to do things to calm them, or change them, or "help" them—this is a big force in psychotherapy. But my work with groups has taught me to have very great respect for people's strengths and potentials and for what people can do for each other in an atmosphere of common inquiry.

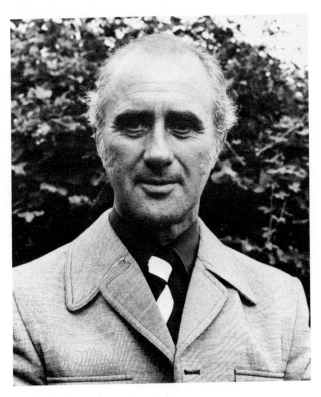

*Robin Skynner, M.B., B.S., M.R.C. Psych., D.P.M.,* is Senior Tutor in Psychotherapy at the Institute of Psychiatry, Great Britain's principal psychiatric training center. He pioneered the development of family therapy in England and has authored numerous articles in this and related areas. His recent book, *One Flesh; Separate Persons,* American edition entitled *Systems of Family and Marital Psychotherapy,* seeks to integrate the contemporary approaches to family and marital therapy.

## A Note on the Type

The text of this book was set, via computer-driven cathode ray tube, in Laurel, an adaptation of Caledonia, a type face originally designed by W. A. Dwiggins. It belongs to the family of printing types called "modern faces" by printers—a term used to mark the change in style of type letters that occurred about 1800. Caledonia borders on the general design of Scotch Modern, but is more freely drawn than that letter.

Composed, printed and bound by Colonial Press Inc.,
Clinton, Massachusetts.
Designed by Virginia Tan